Interviewer's Guide to the Structured Clinical Interview for DSM-IV Dissociative Disorders (SCID-D)

REVISED

Marlene Steinberg, M.D.

Associate Research Scientist
Department of Psychiatry
Yale University School of Medicine
New Haven, Connecticut

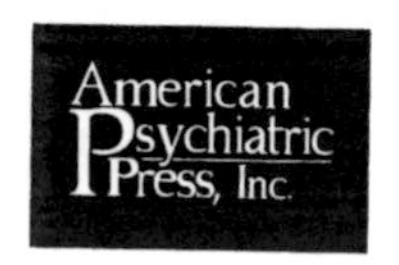

Washington, DC
London, England

Note: The author has worked to ensure that all information in this book concerning drug dosages, schedules, and routes of administration is accurate as of the time of publication and consistent with standards set by the U.S. Food and Drug Administration and the general medical community. As medical research and practice advance, however, therapeutic standards may change. For this reason and because human and mechanical errors sometimes occur, we recommend that readers follow the advice of a physician who is directly involved in their care or the care of a member of their family.

Publications of the American Psychiatric Press, Inc., represent the views and opinions of the individual authors and do not necessarily represent the policies and opinions of the Press or the American Psychiatric Association.

Revised Edition

Manufactured in the United States of America on acid-free paper
08 5 4 3

American Psychiatric Association
1000 Wilson Boulevard
Arlington, VA 22209-3901
www.psych.org

Library of Congress Cataloging-in-Publication Data
Steinberg, Marlene, 1953–
Interviewer's guide to the structured clinical interview for DSM-IV dissociative disorders (SCID-D) / Marlene Steinberg. — Rev.
p. cm.
Includes bibliographical references.
ISBN 0-88048-861-1 (alk. paper)
1. Structured Clinical Interview for DSM-IV Dissociative Disorders—Handbooks, manuals, etc. I. Title.
[DNLM: 1. Dissociative Disorders—diagnosis. 2. Interview, Psychological—methods. 3. Psychiatric Status Rating Scales. WM 173.6 S819i 1994]
RC553.D5S733 1994
616.85′ 23075—dc20
DNLM/DLC
for Library of Congress

94-40649
CIP

British Library Cataloguing in Publication Data
A CIP record is available from the British Library.

Contents

Acknowledgments

This research was supported in part by National Institute of Mental Health First Independent Research Support and Transition Award MH43352 and the Browne-Coxe Research Grant from Yale University School of Medicine.

I gratefully acknowledge Domenic Cicchetti, Ph.D., and Bruce Rounsaville, M.D., for their collaboration with the SCID-D field trials and for their methodological consultation to the *Interviewer's Guide to the SCID-D.* I also thank Drs. Christine Amis, Boris Astrachan, Suzette Boon, Elizabeth Bowman, Etzel Cardeña, Philip Coons, John Docherty, Nel Draijer, Catherine Fine, David Fink, Pamela Hall, Francine Howland, Richard Kluft, George Mahl, Morton Reiser, David Spiegel, Robert Spitzer, and Janet Williams. Likewise Josephine Buchanan, project coordinator for SCID-D research, and the SCID-D staff: Jean Bancroft, Aysha Corbett, Susan Davis, Regina Graham, Jonathan Lovins, Sue Macary, Gerald Melnick, Geanine Peck, Susan Wharfe, and Karen Zych. Finally, for editorial assistance with the revised version, I thank Betsy Frey, M.Phil., and Pamela Harley, Managing Editor, Books, at American Psychiatric Press.

INTRODUCTION

At a time when the incidence of trauma and dissociative phenomena is receiving increasing recognition, there is a need for systematic assessment to improve diagnostic accuracy and allow for appropriate treatment. Although Dissociative Disorders have been observed from the beginnings of psychiatry, the *Structured Clinical Interview for DSM-III-R Dissociative Disorders* (Steinberg 1985) was the first diagnostic instrument for the comprehensive evaluation of dissociative symptoms and disorders. Newly revised for DSM-IV, the *Structured Clinical Interview for DSM-IV Dissociative Disorders* (SCID-D; Steinberg et al. 1989–1993) is a semistructured interview designed to enable a clinically trained interviewer to assess the nature and severity of dissociative symptoms and to diagnose the presence of Dissociative Disorders.

The SCID-D may be used to assess the nature and severity of dissociative *symptoms* in a variety of Axis I and II psychiatric disorders, including the Anxiety Disorders (such as Posttraumatic Stress Disorder [PTSD] and Acute Stress Disorder), Affective Disorders, Psychotic Disorders, Eating Disorders, and Personality Disorders.

The SCID-D was developed to reduce variability in clinical diagnostic procedures and was designed for use with psychiatric patients as well as with nonpatients (community subjects or research subjects in primary care).

In sum, information obtained from the SCID-D enables the interviewer to

1. Rate the severity of five core dissociative symptoms. These global symptoms are grouped into the following categories: amnesia, depersonalization, derealization, identity confusion, and identity alteration. Definitions of severity are used in rating these symptoms.
2. Make diagnostic distinctions based on DSM-IV criteria for the following Axis I disorders: Dissociative Amnesia, Dissociative Fugue, Depersonalization Disorder, Dissociative Identity Disorder (Multiple Personality Disorder), and Dissociative Disorder Not Otherwise Specified, including a new subtype—Dissociative Trance Disorder. In addition, the SCID-D can be used to diagnose Acute Stress Disorder, a new category of anxiety disorder, criteria for which include the presence of dissociative symptomatology.
3. Comprehensively assess dissociative symptoms in psychiatric patients with various Axis I and Axis II disorders, as well as in nonpatients. The assessment of dissociative symptoms is a major goal of the SCID-D; this is done independently of the diagnosis. The SCID-D can thus be added to the battery of diagnostic tests administered to perform a comprehensive diagnostic evaluation.
4. Conduct clinical trials, family studies, longitudinal follow-up studies, cross-cultural analysis of dissociative symptoms and disorders, and epidemiological studies that assess the extent of dissociative symptoms and disorders in the general population.

The SCID-D records information on the subject's functioning, symptomatology, and intra-interview behaviors characteristic of Dissociative Disorders. The SCID-D begins with an overview of the subject's current functioning and psychiatric history. Utilizing screening questions, it then systematically inquires about specific symptoms. The interviewer is then free to choose among several possible follow-up sections, each of which explores the extent of identity disturbance. Many questions are open ended (allowing subjects to elaborate on their symptoms) and are worded specifically for the detection of Dissociative Disorders.

Intra-interview cues suggestive of dissociative

symptoms and/or disorders are assessed and recorded in a systematic manner after the interview. These cues consist of observed behaviors or experiences that take place during the administration of the interview. Incorporating these cues into the ratings, in addition to the verbal responses, best approximates a *clinical* diagnostic interview while maintaining the consistency of a *structured* interview.

The format of the SCID-D is similar to that of the *Structured Clinical Interview for DSM-III-R* (SCID) developed by Robert L. Spitzer, M.D., Janet B. W. Williams, D.S.W., Miriam Gibbon, M.S.W., and Michael B. First, M.D. (1990). The SCID is a structured clinical interview administered for the evaluation of a variety of DSM-III-R (American Psychiatric Association 1987) psychiatric disorders. The SCID has been field-tested in 500 subjects in a project supported by the National Institute of Mental Health (NIMH). The SCID includes modules for many of the major diagnostic classes in DSM-III-R, including the Mood Disorders, Psychotic Disorders, Psychoactive Substance Use Disorders, and Anxiety Disorders.

However, the SCID does not cover the Dissociative Disorders. Hence, the SCID-D can be incorporated as an optional module and used in conjunction with the SCID, or it can be used alone.

The SCID-D is an 8-part interview consisting of the following sections: Psychiatric History, Amnesia, Depersonalization, Derealization, Identity Confusion, Identity Alteration, Associated Features of Identity Disturbance, and Follow-Up Sections on Identity Confusion and Identity Alteration. Following the interview, the following postinterview ratings are to be completed: Intra-Interview Dissociative Cues, DSM-IV Criteria for Dissociative Identity Disorder and Dissociative Disorder Not Otherwise Specified, and the Summary Score Sheet. Each of the five symptom sections (Amnesia, Depersonalization, Derealization, Identity Confusion, and Identity Alteration) begins by inquiring about the nature and severity of the symptom and ends with questions that rule out the presence of organic exclusionary factors to the Dissociative Disorder in which that symptom is predominant. Fugue is assessed in the Amnesia section because amnesia manifests significantly in fugue episodes.

In contrast to a highly structured interview, the SCID-D is not a yes/no checklist of numerous symptoms that are found in many psychiatric disorders. Rather, the SCID-D is a semistructured clinical interview with open-ended questions that elicit elaborate descriptive responses and allow for follow-ups of endorsed symptoms. In addition, SCID-D questions explore the frequency, course, dysfunction, and distress associated with dissociative symptoms.

PART I

Introduction to the Dissociative Symptoms and Disorders

I. Using the Interviewer's Guide

Before administering the SCID-D, the interviewer should familiarize herself or himself with the contents of this *Guide*, as well as with the SCID-D itself. One section of a sample SCID-D interview, concerning the symptom of depersonalization, is reproduced in Appendix 3 for your convenience. This *Interviewer's Guide* provides an overview of the information necessary to understand dissociative symptoms and disorders and to administer, score, and interpret SCID-D interviews.

The *Guide* is divided into three parts: **Part I** is an introduction to the five core dissociative symptoms assessed by the SCID-D and the five dissociative disorders as defined by DSM-IV. This part of the *Guide* is intended to provide a primary theoretical orientation to the phenomenology of dissociation, as well as a brief history of the SCID-D.

Part II is a comprehensive discussion of the basic features and clinical applications of the SCID-D, together with guidelines for clinical practice related to diagnostic and interviewing technique, feedback and follow-up, and suggestions for further study and training.

Part III includes four specific SCID-D case studies as examples of well-conducted interviews and as illustrations of the various clinical applications of the SCID-D.

Part III is followed by **four appendixes,** which contain 1) decision trees for differential diagnosis of the Dissociative Disorders; 2) the Diagnostic Work Sheets; 3) the "Depersonalization" section of the SCID-D interview, reproduced with an experienced clinician's notations and observations; and 4) a set of questions that are often asked about the SCID-D. The decision trees are included as convenient visual summaries of the process of differential diagnosis presented in the case studies. The Diagnostic Work Sheets and the sample "Depersonalization" section are intended as reference guides. The set of questions and answers has been included as a concise summary of the major features and applications of the SCID-D.

Last, because the clinician can offer hope for full recovery to most patients with dissociative disturbances, accurate diagnosis and proper treatment are genuinely beneficial—to the patient and to the rest of society. We hope that you will find this manual a helpful companion to your use of the SCID-D in clinical practice or research.

II. History of the SCID-D

Development of the SCID-D

The SCID-D was developed in 1984–1985 by Marlene Steinberg, M.D., Associate Research Scientist in the Department of Psychiatry at the Yale University School of Medicine.

Field-testing of the SCID-D was performed in collaboration with Bruce Rounsaville, M.D., and Domenic Cicchetti, Ph.D., experts in diagnostic testing and reliability and validity assessment. Consultation with Robert Spitzer, M.D., allowed early access to revisions of the SCID, as well as further consultation regarding methodological design of the SCID-D field trials. In 1989, Dr. Steinberg received the first grant ever awarded by NIMH for research in the field of Dissociative Disorders. This grant allowed for 3-year field trials of the SCID-D, using five interviewers who were blind to the subjects' initial diagnoses.

As a consultant to the American Psychiatric Association's Work Group to Revise DSM-III and DSM-III-R, Dr. Steinberg contributed findings from SCID-D research that were useful in revising the criteria for the Dissociative Disorders in DSM-III-R and DSM-IV.

Reliability and Validity of the SCID-D

The SCID-D was initially pilot-tested on 48 subjects, indicating good to excellent reliability and validity (Steinberg 1985; Steinberg et al. 1990). Additionally, ongoing field trials have been conducted through the NIMH grant. To date, 350 SCID-D interviews have been administered to subjects with a variety of dissociative and nondissociative disorders. All subjects were interviewed by two of five interviewers blind to referring clinician diagnosis. Analysis of the test-retest reliability (over a 7-day interval) of the SCID-D indicates good to excellent reliability and validity with respect to the five dissociative symptoms and Dissociative Disorders (Steinberg 1989–1992, 1994c). These results have been replicated by Goff et al. (1992) at Harvard University and by Boon and Draijer (1991) in Amsterdam. Researchers using the Dutch translation of the SCID-D in Amsterdam found practically identical symptom profiles for the Dissociative Disorders in their Dutch subjects (Boon and Draijer 1991). Further field trials of the Dutch translation, as well as the Hebrew and Spanish translations of the SCID-D, are under way.

SCID-D research indicates that the Dissociative Disorders present specific profiles with respect to these five symptoms (Steinberg 1994c; Steinberg et al. 1990). This research has shown the existence of qualitative and quantitative differences between the presentation of dissociative symptoms in patients with other disorders and those found in patients with Dissociative Disorders.

For further information about the field trials of the SCID-D, refer to Steinberg 1994c and Steinberg et al. 1990.

From DSM-III-R to DSM-IV

The publication and periodic revision of the *Diagnostic and Statistical Manual of Mental Disorders* (DSM) by the American Psychiatric Association provide standard criteria for clinical diagnosis. It is thus valuable for diagnostic instruments to conform to the current version of DSM. The SCID-D was first developed in 1985 and was designed to evaluate DSM-III-R criteria for the Dissociative Disorders. Early access to DSM-IV criteria allowed for their incorporation into the 1993 and 1994 versions of the SCID-D. Diagnostic assessments obtained with the SCID-D are consistent with the criteria adopted in DSM-IV.

Ongoing Research and Current Applications of the SCID-D

The SCID-D is currently used both in outpatient settings and in hospitals for psychiatric inpatients. The SCID-D can be administered as part of a routine psychiatric battery of tests or given to selected patients suspected of having dissociative symptoms. The SCID-D is also being used in numerous research investigations involving patients with a variety of psychiatric disorders.

A multicenter study was conducted by expert researchers in New Haven (Drs. Marlene Steinberg, Bruce Rounsaville, and Domenic Cicchetti), Philadelphia (Drs. Richard Kluft, Catherine Fine, and David Fink), Indiana (Drs. Elizabeth Bowman and Philip Coons), and New Jersey (Dr. Pamela Hall). Over 120 interviews have been conducted and corated among the four sites. Preliminary findings from three of the four sites indicate good to excellent reliability and discriminant validity of the SCID-D for the five Dissociative Disorders and for the SCID-D as a tool for the evaluation of dissociative symptoms encountered within nondissociative syndromes.

In addition, the SCID-D has been translated into numerous languages, including Spanish, Hebrew, Dutch, and Norwegian. These translations will allow for cross-cultural investigation of dissociative symptoms and disorders.

III. Overview of the Dissociative Disorders

The Dissociative Disorders are a group of related disorders with symptoms reflecting a disturbance in the integrative functions of memory, consciousness, and/or identity. There are five Dissociative Disorders whose diagnostic criteria and associated features are extensively described in DSM-IV: Dissociative Amnesia, Dissociative Fugue, Dissociative Identity Disorder (Multiple Personality Disorder), Depersonalization Disorder, and Dissociative Disorder Not Otherwise Specified. Dissociative Disorders newly proposed for DSM-IV are discussed at the end of this section. Although Acute Stress Disorder has been classified as an Anxiety Disorder in DSM-IV, clinicians should note that Criterion B for this disorder specifies the presence of three or more dissociative symptoms during or following the person's experience of severe trauma.

Dissociative Disorders are currently thought to be more common than was originally believed. One significant problem in the diagnosis of the Dissociative Disorders is that isolated symptoms may mimic a spectrum of psychiatric conditions, including Psychotic, Affective, and Personality Disorders (Braun and Sachs 1985; Coons 1984; Kluft 1984, 1987a; Putnam et al. 1986; Rosenbaum 1980). Dissociative Disorders often go undetected for years and are misdiagnosed as other illnesses, such as Depression and Schizophrenia.

In addition to the mimicking of nondissociative symptoms, the elusive nature of dissociative symptoms also contributes to the diagnostic problem. Subjects may be amnestic for their amnesia, may be habituated to their depersonalization, or may present with other symptoms that are easier to describe or that are less likely to be labeled "crazy" (Davison 1964; Kluft 1988; Steinberg 1991). These difficulties underscore the need for a systematic instrument that can detect dissociative symptoms and disorders in a comprehensive way.

One important factor that has prompted the reassessment of the prevalence of the Dissociative Disorders has been the increased recognition of the pervasiveness of child abuse. Research indicates that dissociative symptoms are posttraumatic (Fine 1990; Kluft 1985; Spiegel 1991; Terr 1991). Studies have noted histories of abuse in 72%–98% of all reported cases of the Dissociative Disorders (Kluft 1988; Putnam et al. 1986) and in 50%–75% of general psychiatric patients (Bryer et al. 1987; Ellerstein and Canavan 1980; Emslie and Rosenfelt 1983; Husain and Chapel 1983; Myers 1991; Rosenfeld 1979; Sansonnet-Hayden et al. 1987).

1. Dissociative Amnesia

Dissociative Amnesia is a common Dissociative Disorder and is regularly encountered in hospital emergency rooms (Nemiah 1989). Dissociative Amnesia is typified by the inability to recall important personal information (American Psychiatric Association 1987). The forgotten information is usually of a traumatic nature. The amnesia must be too extensive to be explained by ordinary forgetfulness and must not be due to substance use, such as alcoholic blackout, or a general medical condition, such as seizure disorder, or to the activities of alter personalities (i.e., Dissociative Identity Disorder). There must also be clinically significant distress and/or impairment. Dissociative Amnesia is often seen in wartime and in the victims of single severe traumas such as automobile accidents, witnessing a murder, or natural disasters.

The precipitating trauma for Dissociative Amnesia is most typically a single psychosocial stressor, whereas Dissociative Identity Disorder most commonly presents as the cumulative sequelae of ongoing severe abuse or trauma (Coons and Milstein 1992). In organic amnesia, one's name is commonly the last item to which orientation is lost, and the full return of memory occurs gradually, if at all.

2. Dissociative Fugue

Dissociative Fugue involves sudden, unplanned wandering from home or work, with the assumption of a new partial or complete identity, or confusion about personal identity (American Psychiatric Association 1994). The patient will remain alert and oriented, yet be amnestic for the former identity. *The sophisticated social adaptation distinguishes Dissociative Fugue from fugues seen in organic disorders.* The disorder is distinguished from Dissociative Amnesia by unexpected travel in connection with the amnesia. The disorder is distinguished from Dissociative Identity Disorder by the sudden onset, the presence of a single severe stressor or trauma, and the lack of recurrently appearing complete alter personalities. Unlike Dissociative Identity Disorder, Dissociative Fugue usually consists of a single episode without recurrence, and recovery is usually spontaneous and rapid. For the diagnosis to be made, the fugue symptoms cannot occur as part of Dissociative Identity Disorder or a substance-induced disorder, or as a result of a general medical condition, and must be accompanied by significant distress.

3. Dissociative Identity Disorder

Dissociative Identity Disorder (Multiple Personality Disorder) is the most chronic and severe manifestation of dissociative processes (Kluft et al. 1988). Dissociative Identity Disorder is believed to follow severe and persistent sexual, physical, or psychological child abuse (American Psychiatric Association 1987; Braun and Sachs 1985; Coons et al. 1988; Fine 1990; Kluft 1985; Loewenstein et al. 1987; Putnam 1985; Stern 1984; Wilbur 1984). In this disorder, separate coherent personalities exist within one individual that may control behavior or attitudes, leading to internal struggle and confusion over issues of personal identity. Dissociative Identity Disorder involves inability to recall personal information that is too extensive to be due to normal forgetfulness. The patient will often remain amnestic for periods when an alter identity emerges. In some cases, however, the patient may be able to hold conversations with and otherwise interact internally with an alter personality in much the same way that one would interact with another person. Amnesia between personality states can vary (Kihlstrom 1992; Kluft 1987a); however, some amount of pathological amnesia is almost always present. A person can receive a diagnosis of Dissociative Identity Disorder if his or her suspected symptoms are not due to a Substance-Related Disorder or Schizophrenia.

Dissociative Identity Disorder may mimic a spectrum of psychiatric conditions, including the Psychotic, Affective, and Personality Disorders (Bliss 1980; Braun and Sachs 1985; Coons 1984; Greaves 1980; Kluft 1984, 1987a; Putnam et al. 1986). Patients may experience hallucinations and endorse first-rank symptoms, which contribute to confusion with Schizophrenia (Bliss 1980, 1986; Kluft 1984, 1987a; Rosenbaum 1980; Ross and Norton 1988); depressive symptoms, which contribute to confusion with Affective Disorders (Bliss 1986; Coons 1984; Kluft 1985, 1987a; Marcum et al. 1986; Putnam et al. 1986); and a chaotic life-style, which contributes to confusion with Borderline Personality Disorder (Clary et al. 1984; Horevitz and Braun 1984). People with Dissociative Identity Disorder often receive many misdiagnoses before being diagnosed correctly. Previous diagnoses for patients eventually diagnosed with Dissociative Identity Disorder include Depression, 70%; Neurotic Disorder, 55%; Personality Disorder, 46%; Schizophrenia, 44%; Substance Abuse, 20%; and Bipolar Disorder, 18% (Putnam et al. 1986). The time elapsed between entry into the mental health care system and eventual correct assessment of and beginning of treatment for a patient with Dissociative Identity Disorder may exceed a decade.

4. Depersonalization Disorder

Depersonalization Disorder involves persistent or recurrent experiences of severe depersonalization that lead to distress or dysfunction. The symptom of depersonalization is the feeling that one's body or self is unreal. Individuals may see their body from a distance, feel like they are living in a dream or movie, or feel numb, invisible, or dead. Chronic depersonalization is commonly accompanied by derealization—the feeling that features of the environment are unreal. A patient suffering from Depersonalization Disorder will retain intact reality testing. For a diagnosis of Depersonalization Disorder to be made, the depersonalization must occur independently of Schizophrenia, Dissociative Identity Disorder, or a Substance-Related Disorder and must be accompanied by significant distress or impairment.

Depersonalization as an isolated symptom also appears within the context of a wide variety of major psychiatric disorders (Brauer et al. 1970; Noyes et al. 1977; Steinberg 1991). Rare, mild episodes of depersonalization in college students without a psychiatric illness have been reported following alcohol use, sensory deprivation, mild social or emotional stressors, and sleep deprivation and as a side effect of medications (Roberts 1960; Trueman 1984). Depersonalization Disorder is considered if the symptom of depersonalization is severe and if it is the predominant symptom.

5. Dissociative Disorder Not Otherwise Specified

Dissociative Disorder Not Otherwise Specified (DDNOS) covers syndromes that do not fully satisfy criteria for the other Dissociative Disorders. There are two types of DDNOS: 1) cases that are similar to Dissociative Identity Disorder (but lacking amnesia or complete or distinct personalities), and 2) dissociative syndromes that simply do not fit into any of the other Dissociative Disorder categories. DDNOS includes variants of Dissociative Identity Disorder in which personality "states" may take over consciousness and behavior but are not sufficiently distinct, and variants of Dissociative Identity Disorder in which there is no amnesia for personal information. Other forms of DDNOS include Dissociative Trance Disorder (a cross-cultural category new to DSM-IV), derealization unaccompanied by depersonalization, and dissociative states in people who have undergone intense coercive persuasion (e.g., brainwashing, kidnapping). Refer to the optional "Feelings of Possession" follow-up section in the SCID-D.

Changes in DSM-IV

As mentioned earlier, the SCID-D has incorporated revisions of DSM-III-R, as found in DSM-IV. Two proposed disorders in DSM-IV are Dissociative Trance Disorder and Acute Stress Disorder. Dissociative Trance Disorder was added as a subset of DDNOS to accommodate syndromes that commonly occur in non-Western societies, in which the disorder is not part of a religious ceremony, and leads to distress or dysfunction. Acute Stress Disorder was added to account for cases similar to Posttraumatic Stress Disorder, where there is trauma, followed by a brief period (less than 4 weeks) of anxiety and dissociative experiences that are accompanied by distress or dysfunction.

The organization of the SCID-D allows the clinician to evaluate these newly categorized disorders. Many of the criteria for the new disorders involve questions that are typically asked in the course of the SCID-D interview, and others are found in follow-up sections. For example, Acute Stress Disorder can be evaluated by assessing the severity of dissociative symptoms and by taking into account questions about onset and duration that are included in the assessment of all of the symptoms. Dissociative Trance Disorder can be assessed in the same way, and, additionally, the clinician will find questions dealing specifically with possession and culture-specific rituals in the follow-up sections.

The SCID-D assesses symptoms independent from syndromes. Furthermore, the SCID-D examines different *forms* of the same symptom, as well as associated features and the chronicity of each symptom. In this way, a broad picture of the subject's dissociative experiences can be elicited, and the existence of dissociative symptoms or disorders, past or present, can be assessed.

Summary

The Dissociative Disorders represent different forms of severe dissociation, arising from early childhood or adulthood trauma. The five main disorders can be distinguished from one another and from Acute Stress Disorder by the timing and the nature of the precipitating stressor, chronicity, symptom severity, and, most important, the characteristic constellations of the core dissociative symptoms.

The SCID-D assesses fundamental units of dissociative symptomatology and takes an integrative view of the subject's experiences. It yields a rich resource that can be drawn from to compare the subject's experiences with DSM-IV criteria for a particular Dissociative Disorder.

IV. The SCID-D Dissociative Symptoms

The SCID-D groups dissociative experiences into five global categories, representing the major types of dissociative symptoms. These are amnesia, depersonalization, derealization, identity confusion, and identity alteration. These categories are discrete but interdependent. Additionally, such a conceptualization facilitates the differential diagnosis of the Dissociative Disorders, by stressing symptoms that become predominant in a particular disorder. These symptoms are considered "core," or "primary," because they are considered to be fundamental parts of the process of dissociation; they are not epiphenomena of dissociative processes (such as depression, anxiety, or hallucinations), and each is multifaceted.

Figure 1 is an illustration of the relationship among the five core dissociative symptoms and others that may be endorsed by patients with a Dissociative Disorder.

The symptom of *amnesia* may be defined as a

FIGURE 1. Internal and external manifestations of dissociation.
Source. Reprinted from Steinberg M: *Handbook for the Assessment of Dissociation: A Clinical Guide.* Washington, DC, American Psychiatric Press, 1995. Used with permission.

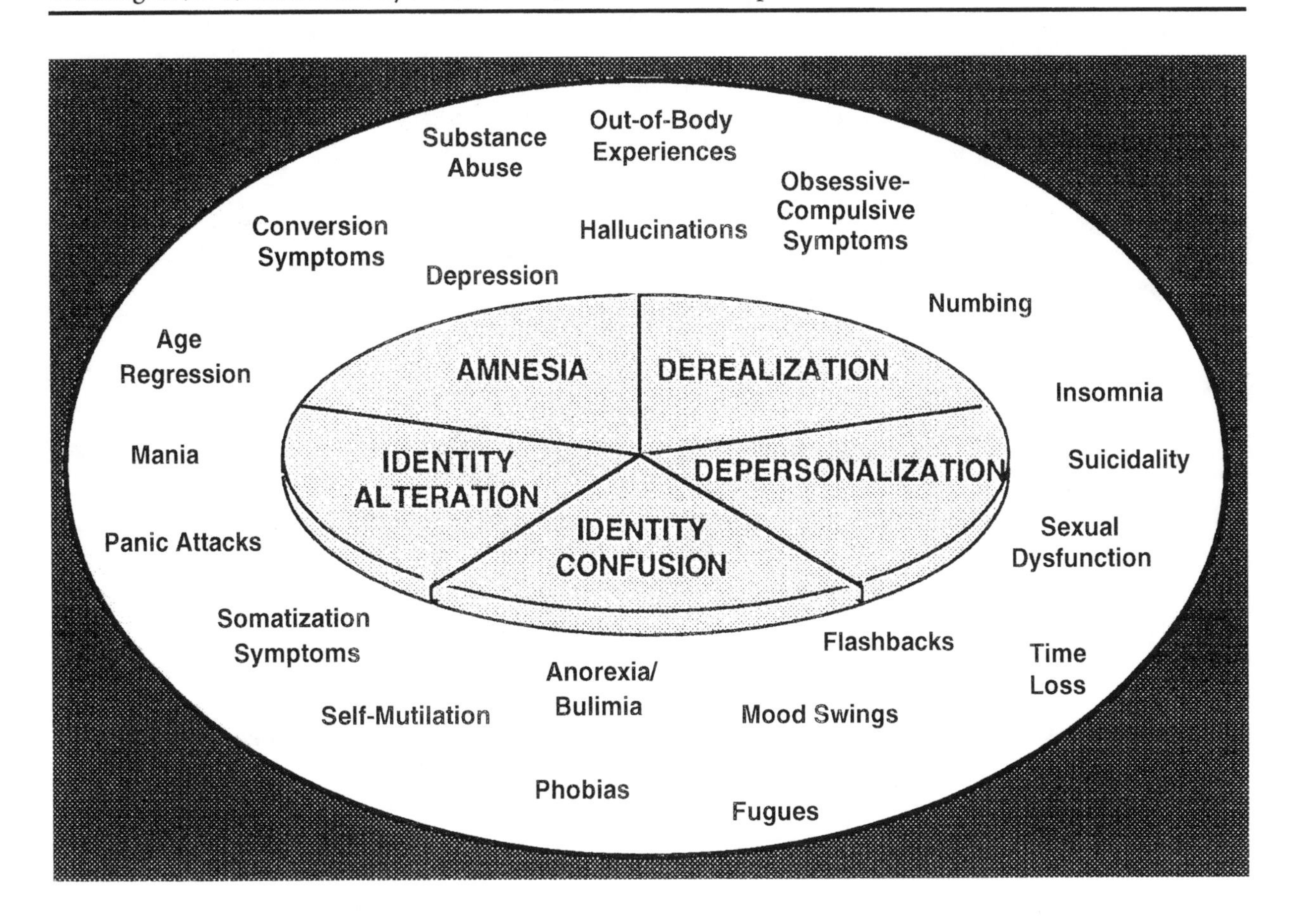

specific and significant segment of time that cannot be accounted for by memory (Steinberg 1985; Steinberg et al. 1990). Amnesia can be classified as the loss of memory for all of a circumscribed period of time (localized amnesia), segments of a circumscribed period of time (selective amnesia), events from a specific time until the present (continuous amnesia), or the loss of memory for one's entire life (generalized amnesia) (American Psychiatric Association 1987, p. 274).

It is even possible for patients to be amnestic for their amnesia, as the following exchange illustrates:

> *Interviewer:* In the past year, how often has it occurred that you couldn't remember, let's say, what has happened to you for days or for weeks?
> *Patient:* I don't know if I can answer that. I really don't, because I don't know how many times that I didn't remember.
> *Interviewer:* That's hard to remember.
> *Patient:* Yes it is. It's just hard to remember how many times I've forgotten.
> (SCID-D interview, unpublished transcript)

Amnesia that occurs in Dissociative Disorders is psychogenic in nature. If a subject interviewed with the SCID-D reports severe amnesia but also reports that this amnesia occurs *only* in the context of drug or alcohol use (such as when smoking marijuana), or if the amnesia is related to brain trauma or organic brain dysfunction, then the diagnoses of Dissociative Amnesia and Dissociative Fugue are excluded. Etiologically, amnesia found in the Dissociative Disorders results from the need to isolate memories connected to traumatic events.

Amnesia occurs across a spectrum, ranging from isolated episodes of minor forgetfulness in subjects without psychiatric disorders to recurrent and persistent inability to recall basic personal information in patients with Dissociative Disorders. Table 1 illustrates the spectrum of amnesia, as measured by the SCID-D.

TABLE 1. The spectrum of amnesia on the SCID-D

DID and DDNOS	Nondissociative and Personality Disorders	No psychiatric disorder
Recurrent to persistent episodes	Isolated episodes	No episodes to isolated episodes
Gaps for hours to years	Rare memory gaps; forgetfulness of a minor nature	Minor forgetfulness associated with stress
Associated with fugues	No fugues	No fugues

Note. DID = Dissociative Identity Disorder. DDNOS = Dissociative Disorder Not Otherwise Specified.
Source. Reprinted from Steinberg M: *Handbook for the Assessment of Dissociation: A Clinical Guide.* Washington, DC, American Psychiatric Press, 1994. Used with permission.

Depersonalization involves detachment of consciousness from the self or from the body. Salient features include a feeling of "strangeness" or unfamiliarity regarding the self and body, a sense that one is observing oneself from the outside, detachment from emotions (numbness, robotic feeling), the feeling that one is living a dream, and other body perception hallucinations such as the feeling that one's body or parts of one's body are missing. Features associated with depersonalization can involve perceptions of parts of the body changing in size, engaging in implausible actions (such as floating, flying, or splitting into two persons), and other manifestations. Although depersonalization may resemble hallucinatory experiences such as those that occur in psychotic disturbances, depersonalization experiences are perceived as occurring "internally." The patient does not attribute the experience to the outside world or believe that the experience can be observed by others. Also, depersonalization is described in "as if" terms, with intact reality testing. Depersonalization in patients with Dissociative Disorders is frequently accompanied by the diagnostically distinguishing feature of ongoing dialogues between the participating and observing selves (Steinberg 1991). These dialogues can be silent or spoken out loud and often involve a struggle.

A patient diagnosed with Dissociative Disorder Not Otherwise Specified endorsed a typical internal dialogue between her participating and observing selves:

> Yeah, I do [the dialogue] like this: *I watch* and I say, "You stupid jerk, you idiot, what are you doing, you can't even do nothing, you could do it before." I mean I think this and *I'm watching myself.* It's like, "Who are you, where did you go to?" (SCID-D interview, unpublished transcript)

The spectrum of depersonalization as measured by the SCID-D is illustrated in Table 2. Also consult Table 6 (p. 23) for additional descriptions of the distinctions between normal and pathological depersonalization.

Derealization, the third symptom assessed by the SCID-D, is defined as a sense that one's surroundings are unreal. This may involve a feeling that one's home or workplace is unfamiliar or a sense that friends or relatives are strange, unfamiliar, or unreal. Derealization is a phenomenal experience of strangeness, which usually occurs in the presence of relevant memories and with the cognitive recognition of that object, person, or event that is experienced as unreal. An individual with derealization may also experience distortions in his or her perception of space or time.

One patient with Dissociative Identity Disorder described her experience of derealization as follows:

> Back then, when I was starting to get better, I would often find myself in my house and have all of the rooms seem very unfamiliar. This isn't where I live. These things aren't mine. I would also have my children and my husband—I knew who they were supposed to be, but they didn't seem familiar at all. And that would last sometimes a couple of days, a week maybe. (SCID-D interview, unpublished transcript)

Table 3 depicts the range of symptoms of derealization, as measured by the SCID-D.

The final two symptoms, identity confusion and identity alteration, are defined specifically for the purposes of the SCID-D. The operationalization of these two concepts allows the SCID-D to systematically assess dissociative disturbances in identity. These concepts have been defined variously by a number of theorists and are presented here with operationalized severity ratings, facilitating systematic assessment.

The symptom of *identity confusion* is defined as a subjective feeling of uncertainty, puzzlement, or conflict about one's identity. This is often accompanied by a struggle as to who one is, or an inner battle regarding identity and decisions. Identity confusion in Dissociative Disorders is different from the iden-

TABLE 2. The spectrum of depersonalization on the SCID-D

DID and DDNOS	Nondissociative and Personality Disorders	No psychiatric disorder
Recurrent to persistent	No episodes to few episodes	No episodes to few episodes
Depersonalization questions elicit descriptions of identity confusion and alteration	No spontaneous elaboration	See Table 6 (p. 23)
Includes interactive dialogues between individual and depersonalized self	No interactive dialogues	No interactive dialogues

Note. DID = Dissociative Identity Disorder. DDNOS = Dissociative Disorder Not Otherwise Specified.
Source. Reprinted from Steinberg M: *Handbook for the Assessment of Dissociation: A Clinical Guide.* Washington, DC, American Psychiatric Press, 1994. Used with permission.

TABLE 3. The spectrum of derealization on the SCID-D

DID and DDNOS	Nondissociative and Personality Disorders	No psychiatric disorder
Recurrent derealization	Few derealization episodes	No episodes to few episodes
Occurs with respect to parents, home, friends	Rarely occurs for family and home	Brief episodes linked to stress
Associated with amnesia and identity alteration	Not associated with amnesia or identity alteration	Not associated with amnesia or identity alteration
Associated with flashbacks and age regression	Not associated with flashbacks or age regression	Not associated with flashbacks or age regression
Recurrent disturbances in perceiving the environment	May experience disturbances in experiencing the environment	No disturbances in perceiving the environment

Note. DID = Dissociative Identity Disorder. DDNOS = Dissociative Disorder Not Otherwise Specified.
Source. Reprinted from Steinberg M: *Handbook for the Assessment of Dissociation: A Clinical Guide.* Washington, DC, American Psychiatric Press, 1994. Used with permission.

tity confusion that often occurs in adolescence and mid-life crises because dissociative identity confusion tends to be severe and tends to strike at the core of identity. Normal "identity crises," as well as identity confusion in other psychiatric disorders, are characterized more by difficulties in finding a stable role in society. In Dissociative Identity Disorder (Multiple Personality Disorder), this identity confusion is often related to conflicting personalities.

The typical dissociative description of identity confusion reflects the theme of internal struggle:

> I feel like an amoeba with fifteen thousand different ideas about where it wants to go. And it's like literally being pulled in every direction possible until there's nothing left, and it's like split in half. That's a constant battle. (SCID-D interview, unpublished transcript)

Identity confusion is a symptom that occurs across a spectrum of severity, ranging from an intermittent struggle between good and bad "parts" occurring in the absence of amnesia in Personality Disorders (Boon and Draijer 1991) to persistent internal struggles regarding identity, characterized by ongoing internal dialogues, in Dissociative Identity Disorder and Dissociative Disorder Not Otherwise Specified. Table 4 illustrates the spectrum of identity confusion.

The fifth symptom, *identity alteration,* is defined as objective behaviors that are manifestations of the assumption of different identities or ego states. A variety of behavioral patterns are common consequences of identity alteration, such as referring to oneself by different names, observing that one possesses a learned skill for which one cannot account, and discovering items in one's possession that one is unaware of having acquired. Other behavioral indicators of identity alteration include people calling the subject an incorrect name or the subject being told by others that he or she has been acting like a completely different person. A subject with identity alteration may also refer to himself or herself as "we." Dissociative cues during the interview can be examined to assess the extent of identity alteration. Severe mood change (especially if accompanied by amnesia), change of voice, and other cues during the interview may indicate identity alteration.

One patient described feedback from others regarding changes in affect and the use of different names as her first indications of this symptom:

Um, they've said to me—the people who don't know that there are any problems at all have said to me, you know, they've made comments about meetings that I've gone to, they've asked me why I was so upset on a particular day. Those type of things. I've been in places where people have called me by other names, but I cannot tell you who they are. Um, I've gotten phone calls from people and I always say, "No, you have the wrong number." It wasn't until therapy that I realized that these people do *not* have the wrong number. I have gone over to [my workplace] and have had people call me by a name I don't recognize, and I don't know who they are. (SCID-D interview, unpublished transcript)

Again, the distinction between the minimal manifestations of identity alteration in nondissociative psychiatric disturbances and the moderate-to-severe identity alteration combined with amnesia that occurs in Dissociative Identity Disorder and Dissociative Disorder Not Otherwise Specified is outlined in Table 5.

TABLE 4. The spectrum of identity confusion on the SCID-D

DID and DDNOS	Nondissociative Axis I and II Disorders	No psychiatric disorder
Recurrent to persistent	Mild to moderate	None to mild
Persistent struggle regarding identity	Confusion regarding one's roles; struggle among good and bad parts	Transient episodes related to stress
Ongoing dialogues	No ongoing dialogues	No ongoing dialogues
Occurs with amnesia	Does not occur with amnesia	Does not occur with amesia

Note. DID = Dissociative Identity Disorder. DDNOS = Dissociative Disorder Not Otherwise Specified.
Source. Reprinted from Steinberg M: *Handbook for the Assessment of Dissociation: A Clinical Guide.* Washington, DC, American Psychiatric Press, 1994. Used with permission.

TABLE 5. The spectrum of identity alteration on the SCID-D

DID and DDNOS	Nondissociative and Personality Disorders	No psychiatric disorder
Recurrent to persistent	Absent to mild	Absent to mild
Different names linked to alternate identities with different behaviors and relationships	No use of different names	
No alternate identities	Role changes occur within their control	
Amnesia for different behaviors	No amnesia for behavior	No amnesia

Note. DID = Dissociative Identity Disorder. DDNOS = Dissociative Disorder Not Otherwise Specified.
Source. Reprinted from Steinberg M: *Handbook for the Assessment of Dissociation: A Clinical Guide.* Washington, DC, American Psychiatric Press, 1994. Used with permission.

V. Assessing the Five Dissociative Symptoms

The SCID-D operationalizes the ratings of severity of the five symptoms of amnesia, depersonalization, derealization, identity confusion, and identity alteration by describing the specific behaviors and experiences that indicate the severity of a dissociative symptom. The Severity Rating Definitions, which start on p. 18, refer the interviewer back to interview items that support or refute the presence and severity of each of the five dissociative symptoms for the subject.

Each symptom is placed on a severity hierarchy that ranges from absent, to mild, to moderate, to severe. The severity of each of the five dissociative symptoms is defined in the Severity Rating Definitions in terms of the frequency, duration, presence or absence of precipitating stressors, and distress/dysfunctionality. In using the Severity Rating Definitions, the interviewer should examine the cross-referenced SCID-D items and choose the *most severe* symptoms endorsed by the subject for rating the severity. Consideration of dissociative episodes should be inclusive of the subject's entire lifetime. Judgment of severity involves a careful balancing of quantity and quality of the symptom. Distress and dysfunction are particularly potent indications of severity.

The Severity Rating Definitions and subsequent scoring establish a standard for inclusion of the symptom on the Diagnostic Work Sheets. Symptoms considered to be clinically significant in diagnosis must qualify as moderate to severe. *Mild symptomatology is not pathological.* The diagnosis of each of the Dissociative Disorders requires the presence of a specific pattern of severity as described on the Diagnostic Work Sheets (see Appendix 2).

Summary Score Sheet

The Summary Score Sheet is a concise summary of the presence and severity of the subject's dissociative symptoms and of the presence of a Dissociative Disorder. This is filled out based on the results of the interview and is a useful reference that can provide at a glance a concise summary of the information obtained from the interview (see Appendix 1). Symptoms are rated for severity from 1 to 4, with 1 indicating absent and 4 indicating severe. Severity is gauged in terms of distress, dysfunctionality, frequency, duration, and course of the symptom, with use of the Severity Rating Definitions as a guide.

For example, for the symptom of derealization, "absent" is rated as 1, "mild" as 2, "moderate" as 3, and "severe" as 4—the maximum rating. The overall score for the subject is the sum of all of the numerical severity ratings of the five total symptoms. This total symptom severity score ranges from 5 to 20. A total score of 5 represents no dissociative symptomatology at all, and a total score of 20 represents severe symptomatology for all five of the dissociative symptoms. This system is also useful for graphically representing SCID-D data (see Figure 2A [pp. 24–25] and Figure 3 [p. 51]) and for statistical analysis.

Because "mild" does not imply pathology, total scores slightly greater than 5 do not necessarily imply mental disorder of any kind. Most control subjects, in fact, score slightly higher than 5. Scores close to 20, on the other hand, do suggest pathological dissociation. Cases of Dissociative Identity Disorder (Multiple Personality Disorder) (the most severe of the Dissociative Disorders) are often accompanied by scores of 17–20 and typically score very close to 20.

The presence of a Dissociative Disorder or Acute Stress Disorder is rated after the completion of the severity ratings. The particular diagnosis can be filled out after completion of the Diagnostic Work Sheets. Experienced clinicians may skip the Diagnostic Work Sheets and go right from the symptom profile to the diagnosis.

SEVERITY RATING DEFINITIONS*

OF INDIVIDUAL DISSOCIATIVE SYMPTOMS

1. Amnesia—A specific and significant block of time that has passed but that cannot be accounted for by memory.	**SCID-D items**
MILD	
● Occasional forgetfulness (lasting seconds to minutes) of a minor nature or amnesia for very early childhood.	
MODERATE (ONE OF THE FOLLOWING)	
● Recurrent brief episodes of amnesia (if prolonged amnesia, rate as severe).	1–16
● Frequent difficulty with memory. May be described as "gaps" in memory.	1–16
● Two or more episodes of amnesia or "blank" spells lasting from 30 minutes up to several hours.	3–5
● Up to two "blank spells" or brief amnestic periods during interview.	265
● Frequent loss of time, or time feels discontinuous.	1–16
● Episodes (1–4) of memory difficulties/amnesia that (ONE OF THE FOLLOWING)	
• produce impairment in social or occupational functioning.	21
• are not precipitated by stress.	22
• are prolonged (over 4 hours).	3–5
• are associated with dysphoria.	23
SEVERE (ONE OF THE FOLLOWING)	
● Subject experiences persistent episodes of amnesia (lasting several hours or longer).	3–5
● Subject experiences episodes of amnesia, brief or prolonged (or time feels discontinuous), most of the time.	1–16
● Subject has recurrently found self in a place away from home and is unaware of how or why he/she went there.	7
● Subject experiences an episode of amnesia in which he/she has a large memory gap for a time in his/her life (after age 6).	3–5
● Subject shows inability to recall important personal information that is too extensive to be explained by ordinary forgetfulness.	15–16
● Subject has abilities and/or talents that he/she cannot recall learning, or subject intermittently forgets previous skills (e.g., subject was a skilled pianist for years and states he/she "forgot" how to play the piano).	1–16, 135
● Subject experiences significant intra-interview amnesia (e.g., subject has amnestic episode during interview, becomes disoriented, and is unaware of who he/she is or who the interviewer is).	265
● Frequent (more than 4) episodes of amnesia that (ONE OF THE FOLLOWING)	
• produce impairment in social or occupational functioning.	21
• do not appear to be precipitated by stress.	22
• are prolonged (over 4 hours).	3–5
• are associated with dysphoria.	23

*Note.** The Severity Rating Definitions are not an inclusive list. The purpose of these definitions is to give the rater a general description of the parameters of the spectrum of dissociative symptoms and their severity.

Prepared for use in conjunction with Steinberg M: *Interviewer's Guide to the Structured Clinical Interview for DSM-IV Dissociative Disorders* (SCID-D), Revised. Washington, DC, American Psychiatric Press, 1994.

SEVERITY RATING DEFINITIONS*

OF INDIVIDUAL DISSOCIATIVE SYMPTOMS

2. Depersonalization—Detachment from one's self, e.g., a sense of looking at one's self as if one is an outsider.	**SCID-D items**
MILD	
● Single episode or rare (total of 1–4) episodes of depersonalization that are brief (less than 4 hours) and are usually associated with stress or fatigue.	38–48, 54, 55, 64
MODERATE (ONE OF THE FOLLOWING)	
● Recurrent (more than 4) episodes of depersonalization. (May be brief or prolonged. May be precipitated by stress.)	38–48, 54, 55, 64
● Episodes (1–4) of depersonalization that (ONE OF THE FOLLOWING)	
• produce impairment in social or occupational functioning.	63
• are not precipitated by stress.	64
• are prolonged (over 4 hours).	55
• are associated with dysphoria.	65
SEVERE (ONE OF THE FOLLOWING)	
● Persistent episodes of depersonalization (24 hours and longer).	38–48, 55
● Episodes of depersonalization occur daily or weekly. May be brief or prolonged.	38–48, 54
● Frequent (more than 4) episodes of depersonalization that (ONE OF THE FOLLOWING)	
• produce impairment in social or occupational functioning.	63
• do not appear to be precipitated by stress.	64
• are prolonged (over 4 hours).	55
• are associated with dysphoria.	65

*Note. The Severity Rating Definitions are not an inclusive list. The purpose of these definitions is to give the rater a general description of the parameters of the spectrum of dissociative symptoms and their severity.

Prepared for use in conjunction with Steinberg M: *Interviewer's Guide to the Structured Clinical Interview for DSM-IV Dissociative Disorders* (SCID-D), Revised. Washington, DC, American Psychiatric Press, 1994.

SEVERITY RATING DEFINITIONS*

OF INDIVIDUAL DISSOCIATIVE SYMPTOMS

3. Derealization—A feeling that one's surroundings are strange or unreal. Often involves previously familiar people.	**SCID-D items**
MILD	
● Single episode or rare (total of 1–4) episodes of derealization that are brief (less than 4 hours) and are usually associated with stress or fatigue.	79–86, 92
MODERATE (ONE OF THE FOLLOWING)	
● Recurrent (more than 4) episodes of derealization. (May be brief or prolonged. May be precipitated by stress.)	79–86, 92
● One or few episodes of derealization that (ONE OF THE FOLLOWING)	
• produce impairment in social or occupational functioning.	91
• are not precipitated by stress.	92
• are prolonged (over 4 hours).	86
• are associated with dysphoria.	93
SEVERE (ONE OF THE FOLLOWING)	
● Persistent episodes of derealization (24 hours and longer).	79–86
● Episodes of derealization occur daily or weekly. (May be brief or prolonged.)	79–86
● Frequent (more than 4) episodes of derealization that (ONE OF THE FOLLOWING)	
• produce impairment in social or occupational functioning.	91
• are not precipitated by stress.	92
• are prolonged (over 4 hours).	86
• are associated with dysphoria.	93

*__Note.__ The Severity Rating Definitions are not an inclusive list. The purpose of these definitions is to give the rater a general description of the parameters of the spectrum of dissociative symptoms and their severity.

Prepared for use in conjunction with Steinberg M: *Interviewer's Guide to the Structured Clinical Interview for DSM-IV Dissociative Disorders* (SCID-D), Revised. Washington, DC, American Psychiatric Press, 1994.

Severity Rating Definitions*

OF INDIVIDUAL DISSOCIATIVE SYMPTOMS

4. Identity Confusion—Subjective feelings of uncertainty, puzzlement, or conflict about one's identity.	**SCID-D items**
MILD	
● Single episode or rare (total of 1–4) episodes of confusion and/or uncertainty as to sense of self and/or who one is. Episodes are brief (less than 3 hours) and may be associated with stress.	101–112
● Single episode or rare (1–4) isolated episodes of identity crisis, characterized by uncertainty of one's role. (Often associated with life-stage transition.)	101–112
MODERATE (ONE OF THE FOLLOWING)	
● Recurrent episodes of confusion and/or uncertainty as to sense of self and/or who one is.	101–112
● Recurrent transient internal struggle regarding who one is.	102–103
● Recurrent confusion regarding one's sexual identity.	102–108
● Episodes (1–4) of identity confusion (not limited to adolescent years) that (ONE OF THE FOLLOWING)	
• produce impairment in social or occupational functioning.	110
• are not precipitated by stress.	111
• are prolonged (over 4 hours).	106
• are associated with dysphoria.	112
SEVERE (ONE OF THE FOLLOWING)	
● Persistent internal struggle or uncertainty as to who one is.	102–103
● One or more episodes of complete loss of one's identity (with or without the assumption of a new identity).	11–13, 101–112
● Recurrent episodes associated with dysphoria (not limited to adolescent years).	112
● Frequent (more than 4) episodes of identity confusion (not limited to adolescent years) that (ONE OF THE FOLLOWING)	
• produce impairment in social or occupational functioning.	110
• are not precipitated by stress.	111
• are prolonged (over 4 hours).	106
• are associated with dysphoria.	112

---

*Note. The Severity Rating Definitions are not an inclusive list. The purpose of these definitions is to give the rater a general description of the parameters of the spectrum of dissociative symptoms and their severity.

Prepared for use in conjunction with Steinberg M: *Interviewer's Guide to the Structured Clinical Interview for DSM-IV Dissociative Disorders* (SCID-D), Revised. Washington, DC, American Psychiatric Press, 1994.

SEVERITY RATING DEFINITIONS*

OF INDIVIDUAL DISSOCIATIVE SYMPTOMS

5. Identity Alteration—Objective behavior indicating the assumption of different identities or ego states, much more distinct than different roles.	**SCID-D items**
MILD	
• Subject reports that he/she plays different roles or exhibits different demeanors, but is aware of this, and states that this is under his/her control (subject may refer to this as "acting"). Generally not associated with dysphoria.	113–117, 131
MODERATE (ONE OF THE FOLLOWING)	
• Subject reports alterations in identity (acting like two different people). However, it is unclear whether these identity alterations take control of his/her behavior or it is unclear whether these alterations in identity represent distinct personalities. The alterations in identity are not always in his/her control.	113–117, 234–244
• Subject spontaneously refers to self in first-person plural ("we") or third person ("he/she").	263
• Subject has internal dialogues between different aspects of self, which have unique characteristics such as age, visual appearance, etc.	138–158, 202–211
• INTRA-INTERVIEW CUES of moderate identity alteration, i.e., several of the following: subtle changes in voice, speech, behavior, demeanor, movement characteristics, or general style of responding.	259–272
SEVERE (ONE OF THE FOLLOWING)	
• Subject has experienced alterations in identity representing distinct personalities that appear to take control of his/her behavior.	113–117, 234–244
• Subject has serious indicators of alteration in identity (such as the use of several names).	118–121
• Subject has considered having or has had a sex-change operation.	101–112
• Subject has referred to self by several names, or others have referred to him/her by different names (not only nicknames, and not for antisocial reasons only).	118–121
• Subject has been told frequently that he/she acts like a completely different person or frequently feels as if he/she has led completely different lives and is unaware of why that has occurred.	114–117
• Subject feels as if there are one or more people inside of him/her who influence his/her behavior.	114–117, 124
• Subject feels as if there is a child inside of him/her, which takes control of his/her behavior and/or speech.	113, 212–222
• Subject has a history of spontaneous age regressions.	113, 136, 223–233
• INTRA-INTERVIEW CUES of severe identity alteration, i.e., several of the following: distinct changes in voice, speech, behavior, demeanor, movement characteristics, or general style of responding.	259–272

---

*Note. The Severity Rating Definitions are not an inclusive list. The purpose of these definitions is to give the rater a general description of the parameters of the spectrum of dissociative symptoms and their severity.

Prepared for use in conjunction with Steinberg M: *Interviewer's Guide to the Structured Clinical Interview for DSM-IV Dissociative Disorders* (SCID-D), Revised. Washington, DC, American Psychiatric Press, 1994.

Distinguishing Between Normal and Pathological Depersonalization (Table 6)

Several studies have indicated that depersonalization may occur in normal subjects who are under mild stress (Roberts 1960; Trueman 1984). However, in the Dissociative Disorders, depersonalization tends to be recurrent and persistent and is associated with distress and/or dysfunctionality. SCID-D research has indicated that the distinguishing diagnostic feature of depersonalization in subjects with Dissociative Disorders is ongoing interactive dialogues. To clarify the distinctions between normal and pathological depersonalization, the spectrum of depersonalization is illustrated in Table 6. The table describes increasing severity of symptom levels, moving from left to right. The *left column* summarizes the features of brief, mild depersonalization in the general population. The *middle column* summarizes the characteristics of transient depersonalization that are most often seen in patients exposed to life-threatening danger such as an automobile accident. The *right column* then briefly reviews the salient features of depersonalization in the Dissociative Disorders.

When rating a SCID-D interview, you will have to decide whether the subject's endorsed symptoms of depersonalization are clinically significant. Familiarity with Table 6 will help you use the Severity Rating Definitions to differentiate between depersonalization as an occurrence in everyday life and depersonalization as a symptom of a Dissociative Disorder.

TABLE 6. Distinguishing between normal and pathological depersonalization

	Common mild depersonalization	Transient depersonalization	Pathological depersonalization
Context	Occurs as an isolated symptom	Occurs as an isolated symptom	Occurs within a constellation of other dissociative or nondissociative symptoms *or* with ongoing interactive dialogues
Frequency	One or few episodes	One episode that is transient	Persistent or recurrent depersonalization
Duration	Depersonalization episode is brief; lasts seconds to minutes	Depersonalization of limited duration (minutes to weeks)	Chronic and habitual depersonalization lasting up to many years
Precipitating factors	• Extreme fatigue • Sensory deprivation • Hypnagogic and hypnopompic states • Drug or alcohol intoxication • Sleep deprivation • Medical illness/toxic states • Severe psychosocial stress	• Life-threatening danger. This is a syndrome noted to occur in 33% of individuals immediately following exposure to life-threatening danger, such as near-death experiences and auto accidents (Noyes et al. 1977) • Single, severe psychological trauma	• Not associated with precipitating factors listed in Column 1. • May be precipitated by a traumatic memory. • May be precipitated by a stressful event but occurs even when there is no identifiable stress. • Occurs in the absence of a single immediate severe psychosocial trauma.

SCID-D Symptom Profiles of the Dissociative Disorders (Figure 2A)

Figure 2A shows the profile of dissociative symptoms for the five main DSM-IV Dissociative Disorders. These graphs employ the numerical scaling (1–4) of the severity of dissociative symptoms. It may be useful to refer to this figure in the differential diagnosis of the Dissociative Disorders.

Examine Figure 2A for a moment. The *vertical axes* use both qualitative units (severity description from none to severe) and quantitative units (corresponding score of 1–4). The *horizontal axes* show the five symptom areas. The graphs plot the different patterns made by the typical symptom severities in different Dissociative Disorders. Each *line* forms what is called a "symptom profile" of the disorder.

It should be noted that Acute Stress Disorder

FIGURE 2A. SCID-D symptom profiles of the Dissociative Disorders.

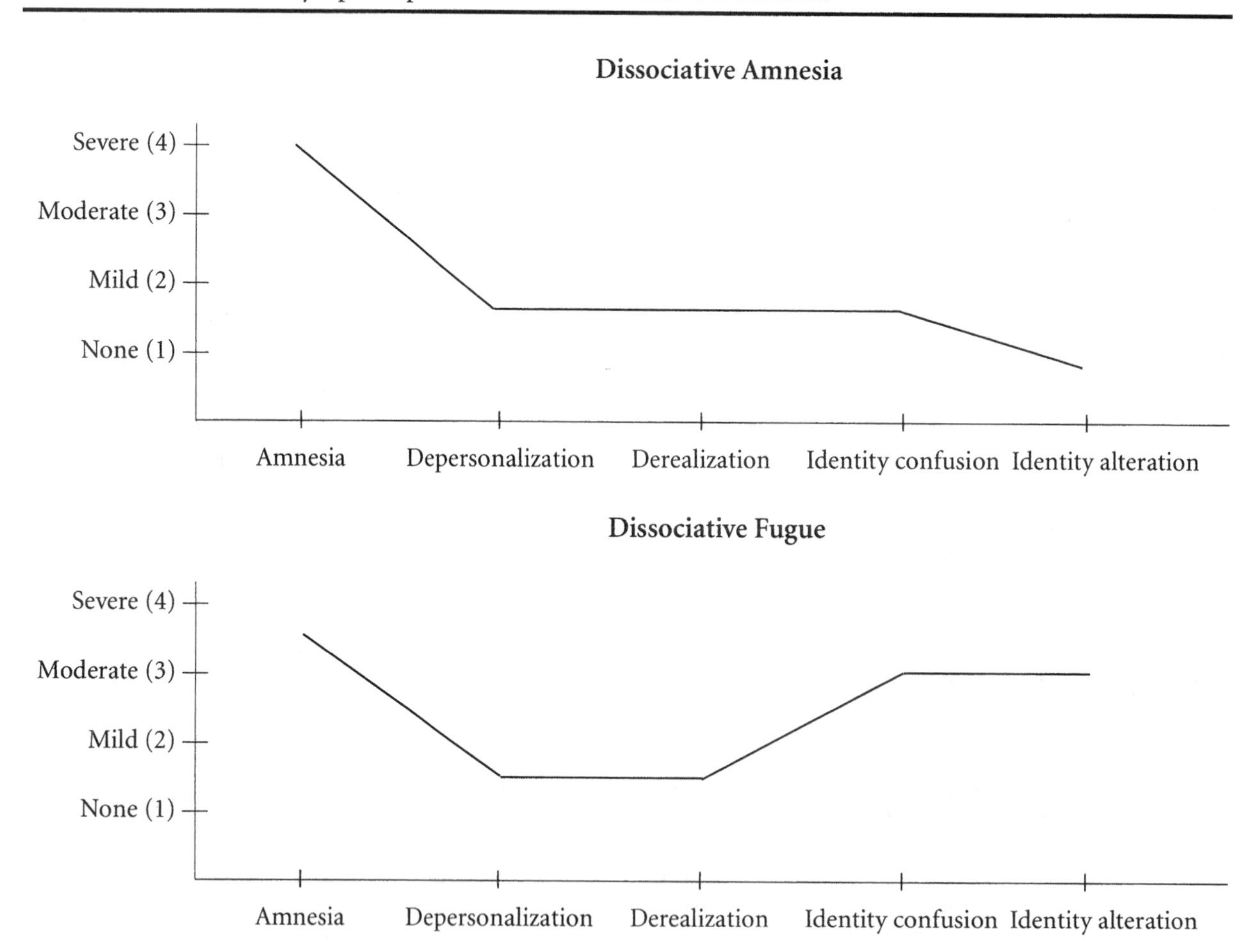

can generate several characteristic profiles, in that Criterion B for this disorder specifies that the person manifest three or more symptoms of depersonalization, derealization, or amnesia. As a result, individuals with Acute Stress Disorder may present with several different combinations of these three core symptoms at a high level of severity, combined with a low or moderate severity level for identity confusion and identity alteration (Figure 2B).

Graphing dissociative symptom scores is a convenient, visual, and systematic way of conveying important information about a person's dissociative symptomatology.

Depersonalization Disorder

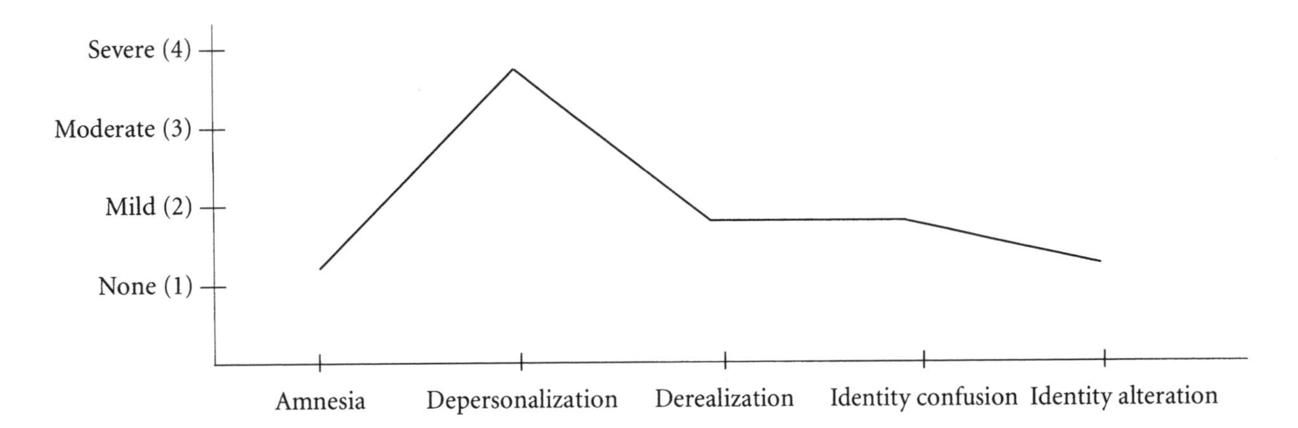

Dissociative Identity Disorder (DID) (Multiple Personality Disorder) and Dissociative Disorder Not Otherwise Specified (DDNOS)

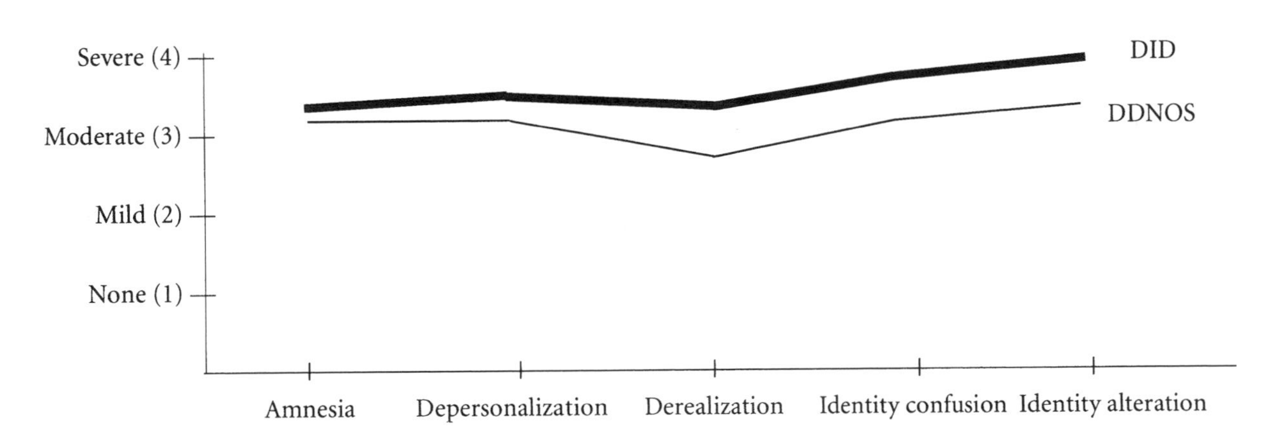

FIGURE 2B. SCID-D symptom profiles for Acute Stress Disorder.

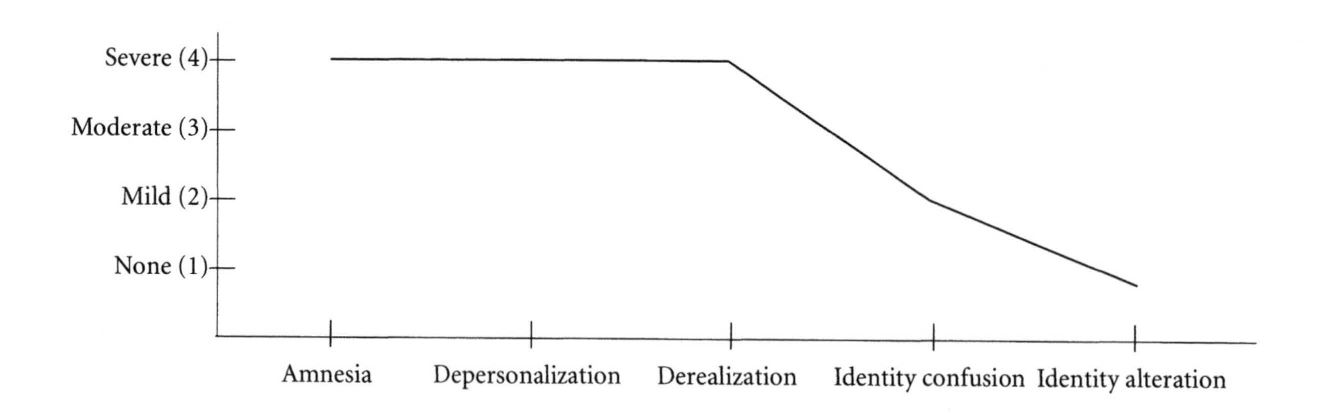

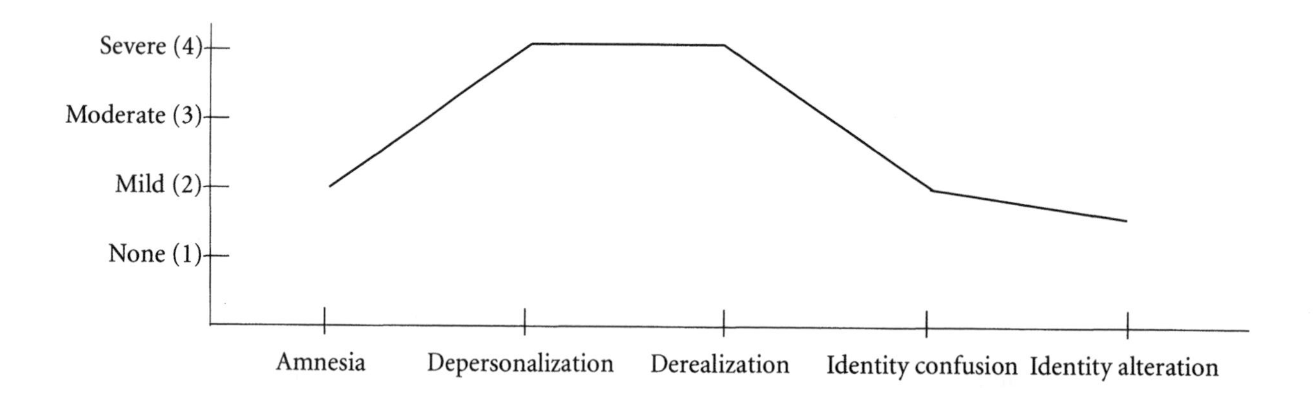

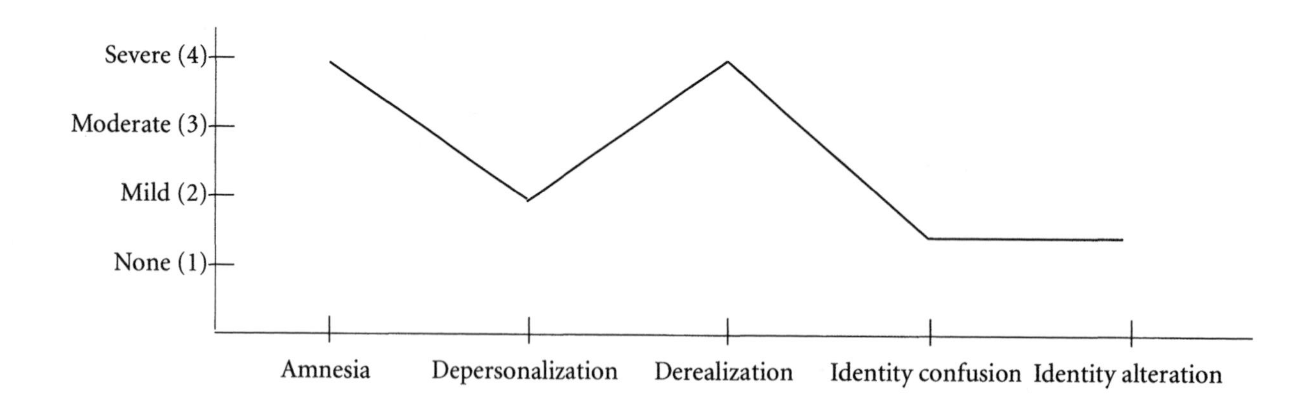

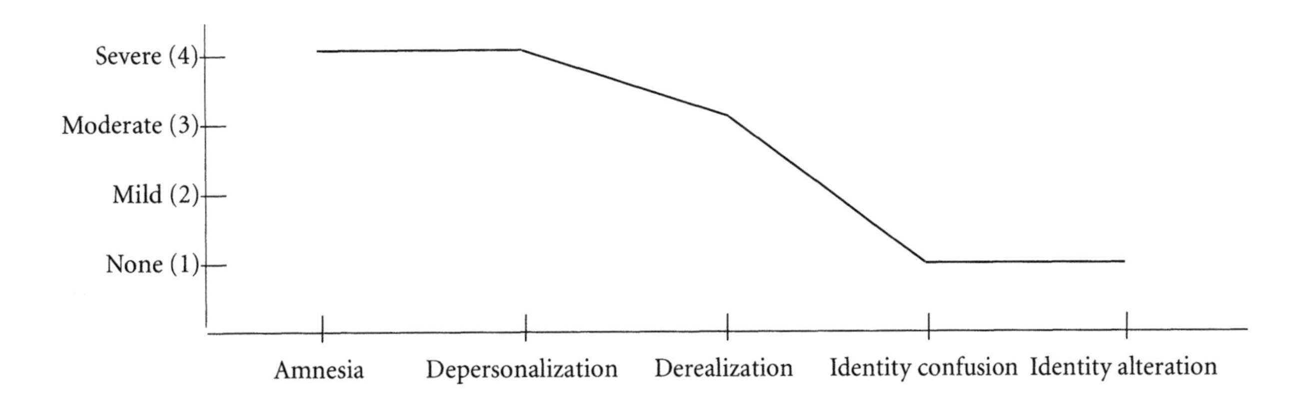

Severe (4)
Moderate (3)
Mild (2)
None (1)
Amnesia
Depersonalization
Derealization
Identity confusion
Identity alteration

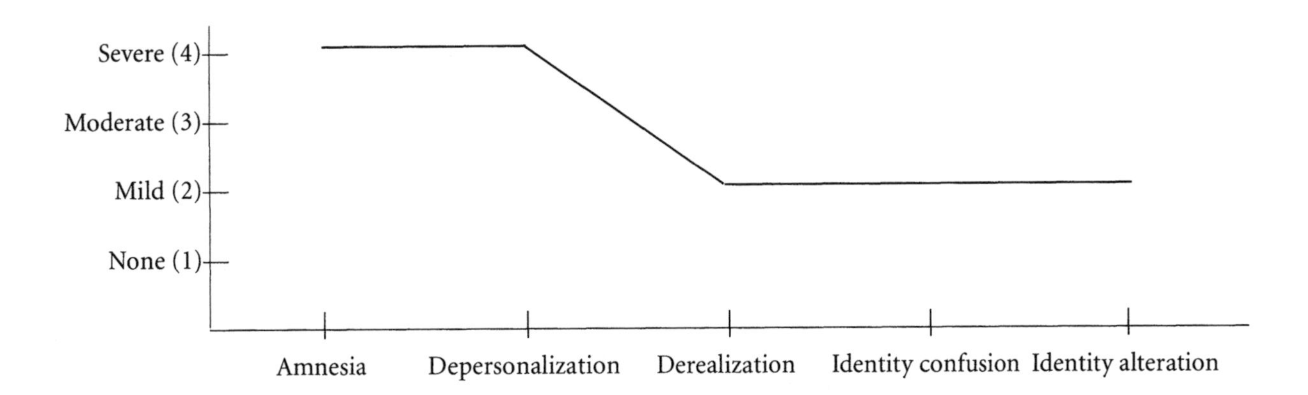

Severe (4)
Moderate (3)
Mild (2)
None (1)
Amnesia
Depersonalization
Derealization
Identity confusion
Identity alteration

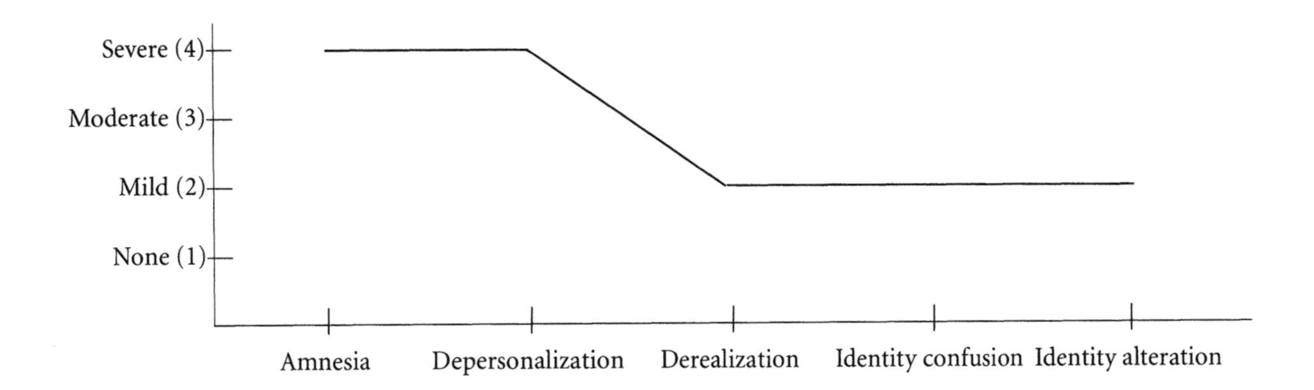

Severe (4)
Moderate (3)
Mild (2)
None (1)
Amnesia
Depersonalization
Derealization
Identity confusion
Identity alteration

PART II

USING THE SCID-D

VI. Clinical Applications and Administration

The SCID-D is a time- and cost-effective instrument with a variety of clinical applications. In addition to its diagnostic utility, it is a tool that can be used for patient education regarding the nature and significance of dissociative symptomatology during a follow-up session with the subject. Chapter XII describes the clinical indications and purposes of follow-up interviews in further detail. Also refer to Case 4 in Chapter XIV for a specific example of the SCID-D's usefulness in patient education. Because the SCID-D's format facilitates long-term monitoring of patients' symptoms, a clinician can administer the instrument at 6-month or yearly intervals to monitor changes in symptomatology and reassess treatment strategy accordingly.

In addition, because the SCID-D is designed to be filed with patients' charts, it provides easily accessible symptom documentation, for record keeping and psychological reports. Cases 2 and 3 in Chapter XIV are included as examples of the type of psychological report that can be compiled from the information acquired in a well-conducted interview. These two cases also illustrate an experienced clinician's use of the SCID-D in planning a course of treatment to meet the specific needs of an individual patient.

Practitioners of hypnosis will find the SCID-D particularly relevant to their work because the instrument allows accurate assessment of the patient's baseline dissociative symptomatology. By its nature, hypnosis involves the induction of controlled dissociation by teaching the patient to concentrate attention in a highly selective fashion. Without the information obtained by prehypnotic assessment of dissociative symptoms, as performed by the SCID-D, a clinician might find it more difficult to ascertain whether symptoms elicited under hypnosis are secondary to the induction or primary to a Dissociative Disorder. Because the SCID-D is intended to be filed with patients' charts, practitioners of hypnosis will have convenient documentation of baseline dissociative symptoms.

Last, the SCID-D is a diagnostic tool that can be helpful to clinicians involved in the assessment of patients who are defendants in legal proceedings, especially in cases in which there is a suspicion of Dissociative Identity Disorder. In the first place, the Summary Score Sheet could be offered in courtroom evidence as a form of symptom documentation. Because Dissociative Identity Disorder complicates evidentiary issues (Lewis and Bard 1991), the SCID-D Interview and Summary Score Sheet provide an additional form of documentation that is less controversial than videotaping, Amytal interviews, or hypnosis. In addition, the SCID-D's good-to-excellent interrater reliability allows for reasonable confidence in findings regarding evaluation of a patient by more than one examiner. In cases in which an accused person must be transferred from one jurisdiction to another, the instrument can be administered repeatedly by different interviewers without prejudice to the accused individual.

Administration of the SCID-D

The SCID-D can be administered during one session; however, a clinician should feel free to schedule two sessions, for example, when interviewing subjects who endorse a large number of symptoms or symptom episodes. The length of the interview depends on the number and complexity of symptoms endorsed. Because this semistructured interview elicits descriptions of experiences, more positive responses may require significantly more interviewing time. For normal subjects, the interview can be completed in less than 30 minutes. For subjects with nondissociative disorders, the time of administration ranges from 30 minutes to 1.5 hours. Subjects with Dissociative Disorders usually require between 40 minutes and 2.5 hours. These subjects should certainly be given enough time to describe their experiences fully.

Although administration of the full SCID-D thus requires 2–3 hours of the interviewer's time, the instrument is actually highly cost-effective in terms of its demonstrated ability to detect previously undiagnosed cases of Dissociative Disorder. Given present figures regarding the average Dissociative Disorder patient's length of time in misdirected therapy before establishment of the correct diagnosis (i.e., 7–10 years; Coons et al. 1988; Kluft 1987a; Putnam et al. 1986), earlier detection of a Dissociative Disorder using the SCID-D allows for rapid implementation of appropriate treatment strategies.

The Interviewer's Preparation and Training

Interviewers should be mental health professionals with clinical experience, knowledge of psychiatric illnesses, and familiarity with DSM-IV diagnostic criteria. Interviewers should also familiarize themselves with the literature on dissociation, as well as this *Interviewer's Guide.* Additional training and/or supervision in the use of the SCID-D is recommended for readers who are new to the field of dissociation.

The SCID-D interview can be administered to psychiatric outpatients, psychiatric inpatients, and normal subjects. The interview can be used to assess the presence of dissociative symptoms in subjects with or without Dissociative Disorders; to screen for the presence of a Dissociative Disorder and if a symptom is present to diagnose it; and to gather data for research purposes. The interview should be administered in a relaxed manner, with respect for the subject's sensitivity about symptom disclosure. Refer to Chapter IX for further discussion of interviewing principles and techniques.

The following additional materials are recommended for obtaining the best results with the SCID-D:

1. Review the systematic assessment of dissociative symptoms and disorders described in *Handbook for the Assessment of Dissociation: A Clinical Guide* (Steinberg 1995). Other recommended readings include

   Tasman A, Goldfinger SM (ed): *American Psychiatric Press Review of Psychiatry,* Volume 10. Washington, DC, American Psychiatric Press, 1991, pp. 139–276. (Five chapters devoted to the assessment and treatment of the Dissociative Disorders are included in this book.)

   Spiegel D: "The Dissociative Disorders," in *The American Psychiatric Press Textbook of Psychiatry,* 2nd Edition. Edited by Hales RE, Yudofsky SC, Talbott JA. Washington, DC, American Psychiatric Press, 1994, pp 633–652

2. Study the *Interviewer's Guide to the Structured Clinical Interview for DSM-IV Dissociative Disorders* (SCID-D), as well as the SCID-D interview itself, the Summary Score Sheet, and the Severity Rating Definitions.
3. If you are unfamiliar with the field of dissociation, you may want to attend SCID-D workshops given on assessment of Dissociative Disorders and symptoms.
4. When you are beginning to learn how to administer the SCID-D, you may find it helpful to administer one section at a time to a subject, focusing on each of the five symptoms separately. Once you have familiarized yourself with each of these sections, you will be prepared to administer the complete interview.
5. Gain experience by administering the SCID-D to subjects with and without Dissociative Disorders to recognize the full spectrum of dissociative symptoms. Initially, you may want to review your practice ratings with a colleague trained in SCID-D administration.

VII. Basic Features

The following features were incorporated into the SCID-D to best approximate a clinical diagnostic interview yet maximize reliability. Questions and issues specific to the Dissociative Disorders are included. Features unique to the SCID-D are indicated with an *asterisk* (*).

1. The interview schedule includes operationalized questions, yet it also allows for maximum flexibility. Like the Schedule for Affective Disorders and Schizophrenia (SADS; Endicott and Spitzer 1978) and the SCID, the SCID-D has preliminary questions that allow the interviewer to decide whether to continue with a subsequent set of questions. If the preliminary question is answered negatively, associated follow-up questions can be skipped. On the other hand, if the preliminary question is answered positively, the interviewer goes on to the related follow-up questions. Spontaneous follow-up questioning is also an important part of the interview.

   There are also nine follow-up sections, which are used to further assess identity confusion and alteration, specifically the severity of these dissociative symptoms. If responses to certain questions are positive, the interviewer has a choice of proceeding to two of the nine follow-up sections for further exploration of the subject's symptoms. The decision as to which follow-up section to enter is individualized for each subject, depending on which follow-up section seems most likely to tap that particular subject's experiences. Those customized "facets" are thus used as entry points into the subject's history of identity confusion and alteration.
2. The interview schedule is arranged so that initial inquiries regarding symptoms are worded in an open-ended manner. This format was chosen to allow subjects maximum flexibility in describing their symptoms, which could not be obtained by merely asking for agreement or disagreement. On a more structured questionnaire or interview, a yes answer from a subject who has misunderstood a question will still be mistakenly scored as a yes. With the SCID-D, the subject is asked for more than an affirmation or negation. For instance, one question in the amnesia section is: "How did it [amnesia] interfere with your social relationships? How did it interfere with your ability to work?" Other questions following direct questions include: "Can you describe that?" "What was that experience like?" "How might a dialogue go?"

   In addition to the subject's explication of his or her experience and the SCID-D follow-up questions, the interviewer uses clinical judgment in asking unscripted follow-up questions, should clarification of the subject's response be necessary. Often the subject finishes his or her description with a comment that seems important to the interview, and the interviewer may then ask, "Could you say more about that?" Allowing the subject to explore his or her past experiences often enhances the vividness of these reports, as well as the subject's ability to recount a greater range of memories, and in more detail than would be possible in a yes/no or multiple-choice format.

*3. The interview schedule contains two types of questions. Questions of the first type ask about the presence or absence of symptoms in a *direct* manner, followed by questions such as, "What is that experience like?" that elicit a description and elaboration of the original positive endorsement. Other questions are worded in an *indirect* manner, by inquiring about associated features of a symptom. Because individuals with Dissociative Disorders may evade answering questions when asked directly (e.g., they are amnestic for the pertinent information, and/or they may defensively withhold information), questions concerning clinically relevant associated symptoms and experiences often facilitate the subject's ability to answer openly. These associated aspects may be more subtle than the overt symptom and may increase the likelihood of detection from the multifacetedness of the symptoms. For instance, one question is "Have you ever felt like a completely different person?" Many subjects will answer no to this question but will answer yes to an associated question like, "Have you ever found things in your possession that seemed to belong to you, but you could not remember how you got them?"

These two strategies also reflect the SCID-D's distinction between *subjective* and *behavioral* manifestations of symptomatology. In many cases, behavioral manifestations may be easier for the subject to report because they may be perceived as unrelated to the symptom itself. Most questions regarding the symptom of identity alteration assess *behavioral* manifestations of the symptom, because amnesia often hinders individuals' subjective awareness of their identity alteration.

*4. Numerous questions allow for a variety of inquiries regarding the same symptom. Several questions regarding one symptom are asked because there is often a multifaceted presentation of the dissociative symptoms. For example, some individuals with depersonalization episodes may experience feeling detached, whereas others may not complain of detachment but rather of seeing themselves outside of their body. Asking both questions allows for a comprehensive and reliable assessment of an episode of depersonalization.

*5. Intra-interview cues suggestive of dissociative symptoms and/or disorders are assessed and recorded in a systematic manner. These cues include body movements and changes in speech or language patterns that occur *during* the interview and that are not directly assessed through administered questions. Incorporating these behaviors and symptoms in conjunction with the verbal responses best approximates a clinical *unstructured* interview and is therefore essential for the comprehensive assessment of the Dissociative Disorders. These dissociative cues are often strong indicators of Dissociative Disorders. They include spontaneous age regression, trancelike appearance, and intra-interview amnesia.

*6. The SCID-D allows the interviewer to record inconsistencies in the subject's responses and to include the presence of inconsistent responses in the overall assessment of the subject. Previous structured interviews forced the interviewer to choose the "best" rating and to decide which of two inconsistent responses was to be rated. These interviews may imply that the interviewer should choose whichever response he or she feels is most valid. On other tests, such as the Minnesota Multiphasic Personality Inventory (MMPI; Hathaway and McKinley 1970), numerous inconsistent responses may lead to invalidation of the score or a sometimes incorrect interpretation that the subject is malingering rather than presenting with actual symptoms. On the SCID-D, the interviewer is able to note that the subject has answered any given question in both the affirmative and the negative and then to record both responses. Thus, the interviewer is not forced to choose the "best" response. The critical clinical rationale underlying this diagnostic strategy is that inconsistent responses are common in individuals with Dissociative Disorders and may, in themselves, represent the discrepant dissociated aspects of the subject's personality.

*7. The interviewer's overall assessment utilizing the SCID-D is based on the interviewer's ratings of the subject's verbal responses, intra-interview dissociative cues, and inconsistent responses. Ratings of verbal responses include the interviewer's clinical assessment of the subject's response to the questions. Thus, overall symptom assessment and diagnosis represents a synthesis of the subject's verbal and nonverbal responses and the interviewer's clinical assessment of inconsistent responses. In this way, the SCID-D incorporates important strengths of a clinical unstructured interview, while preserving the reliability derived from a systematic instrument. The SCID-D is semistructured, with open-ended questions and a flexible design.

*8. The SCID-D offers severity ratings for five symptom areas associated with dissociative pathology, based on the information obtained from the SCID-D. These symptom areas are amnesia, depersonalization, derealization, identity confusion, and identity alteration. Definitions of severity have been developed and are utilized for the rating of these symptoms. (See the SCID-D Severity Rating Definitions, pp. 18–22.) This set of anchored clinician ratings is similar to that in the Raskin Depression Scale (Raskin et al. 1969) and the Global Assessment Scale (Endicott et al. 1976) and may provide additional information for the various diagnostic groups studied. Characteristics indicating severity of a symptom include frequency, duration, and degree of dysphoria and dysfunctionality.

9. The SCID-D's questions incorporate DSM-IV criteria and thus allow for the determination of the presence of an Axis I diagnosis of Dissociative Disorder (lifetime prevalence or a current episode) or Acute Stress Disorder.

*10. The SCID-D is adaptable to future revisions of DSM. The SCID-D contains 277 questions and asks about many different aspects of dissociative experiences. Assessment of symptoms and diagnosis of disorder involves using SCID-D responses as building blocks, which are grouped together with respect to specified criteria, such as those of DSM-IV. Dissociative symptoms are first assessed independently of a particular diagnosis. Categories of dissociative disturbances that were added in DSM-IV (e.g., Dissociative Trance Disorder) can be assessed because the SCID-D asks questions related to these new categories. The SCID-D contains a follow-up section on possession, for instance, that asks about possession experiences and the relation of these to the subject's religion or culture.

VIII. Organization and Scoring

This section describes how the SCID-D is organized and provides instruction as to how the interviewer makes decisions throughout the interview. Instructions regarding final assessment of symptoms and diagnosis are presented in Chapters V and X.

Although the overall format of the SCID-D is based on that of the SCID, several modifications have been incorporated into the SCID-D. The following describes the format of the SCID-D and provides guidance on how to proceed through the sections. Features unique to the SCID-D are indicated below with an *asterisk* (*).

1. Like the SCID, the SCID-D employs a three-column organization. The *left-hand column* includes interview questions, as well as instructions for the interviewer. Instructions include those for skipping specific questions when they are irrelevant to the subject. The *middle column* includes DSM-IV criteria, definitions of symptoms relevant to specific questions, and examples to help clarify ratings. The *right-hand column* contains the codes (or boxes) for rating the questions. At the bottom of each page are displayed the definitions of these rating codes: ? = inadequate information, N = no, Y = yes, and I = inconsistent information. When a question cannot be answered in this yes/no format, the *appropriate* boxes are checked in the middle column. Examples of this type of question include those that inquire about frequency and age at onset of a symptom. An example of this multicolumn format is shown in the box below:

38. Have you ever felt that you were watching yourself from a point outside of your body, as if you were seeing yourself from a distance (or watching a movie of yourself)?	**Depersonalization** "An alteration in the perception or experience of the self so that one feels detached from, and as if one is an outside observer of, one's mental processes or body (e.g., feeling like one is in a dream)" (DSM-IV, p. 766). "Patients feel that their point of conscious 'I-ness' is outside their bodies, commonly a few feet overhead, from where they actually observe themselves as if they were a totally other person" (Nemiah 1989, p. 1042).	? N Y I

? = inadequate information N = no Y = yes I = inconsistent information

2. The initial, general question for each diagnosis included in the SCID-D asks about the presence of a particular symptom. These questions begin by asking, "Have you ever had (felt, etc.) . . . ?" If the subject mentions having had some of these symptoms prior to questioning, the initial question can be skipped, and the follow-up question can be modified by starting the question with, "You mentioned that you have had (felt, etc.) . . . ?"
3. If the subject states that he or she has had the symptom asked about in the initial question, additional, description-seeking questions are asked to explore the nature and frequency of the symptom. The interviewer should record the subject's response in the space provided. This ensures that the interviewer has sufficient information to rate the question. Responses that are very long need not, of course, be recorded in their entirety in the space provided. The interviewer should record a sentence or two that best captures the major contents of the response.
4. Chronicity questions are asked to assess the severity of a symptom. These questions ask, "How often does that occur?"; possible answers are rarely (4 episodes total), occasionally (up to 4 episodes per year), frequently (5 episodes or more per year), monthly (up to 3 episodes per month), daily or weekly (4 episodes or more per month), or unclear (subject cannot answer sufficiently [often associated with memory difficulty]). Other questions ask about duration, age at onset, and most recent episode.
5. When referring to a symptom that the subject has endorsed, the interviewer individualizes the question by using the subject's *own words* to refer to that symptom. For instance, suppose the subject answers positively to a question about derealization by stating, "It seemed as if my dog was like a cartoon character." To determine the frequency of this symptom, the interviewer is instructed to ask, "How often have you had ______________________?"
   [endorsed symptoms of derealization]

   The interviewer should complete this question using the subject's own description of the derealization episode (seeing his dog as a cartoon character). This ensures that both the interviewer and the subject are referring to the same thing and that the subject is not baffled or misled by erudite lingo.
6. There are numerous questions that include instructions to the interviewer. These instructions are written in *capital letters.* Examples are single or the first of multiple follow-up questions (e.g., "IF YES: What was that experience like?").
7. Questions in *parentheses* are optional and may be asked if further clarification or elaboration of the subject's response seems necessary. Questions *not in parentheses* should be asked of each subject. Nevertheless, there are numerous occasions in the interview where the interviewer is given the option of skipping a series of questions. This is done so that time is not spent exploring information that is irrelevant to the interview. Naturally, if the subject answers negatively for a question, the questions that follow prefaced by "IF YES" should be skipped. At certain points, preliminary questions allow the interviewer to skip a series of questions about one symptom that is not endorsed. At other points, these "decision" questions allow the interviewer to end a line of questioning that is not obtaining positive responses.
8. Each question, unless otherwise specified, is coded utilizing the following standard ratings:

   ? = inadequate information. This indicates that the information given is inadequate to rate the item as N or Y. A rating of ? may be used when the subject answers by stating, "I don't know," and attempts at clarification fail to elicit sufficient information to rate the response as yes or no.

   N = no. This rating indicates that the symptom or experience described in the question is clearly absent or has never occurred.

Y = *yes.* This rating indicates that the symptoms or experiences described in the specific question have been or are present in the person's life.

*I = *inconsistent information.* This rating indicates that the interviewer has obtained from the subject inconsistent or discrepant information regarding the symptoms or experiences described in the question. Rather than attempting to choose which of the differing responses are "more valid," the interviewer notes that inconsistent information was obtained by using a rating of I. The following are examples of inconsistent answers receiving a rating of I:

> A subject denies hallucinations but is observed to talk to himself and appears to be responding to voices.
>
> A subject nods her head (as if to say yes) in response to a specific question, yet verbally responds by saying "No."
>
> A subject denies having had a depersonalization episode, although earlier in the interview that subject described having had a depersonalization episode.

When using the rating of I, the interviewer should note both of the responses that were inconsistent with each other. In the latter example, for instance, the interviewer would rate the response in the following manner:

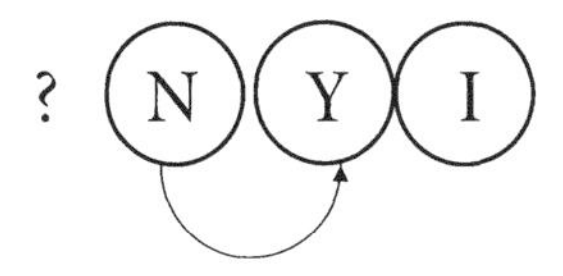

This rating informs us that the subject responded to the questions with an inconsistent response (rating of I), that the subject stated that the symptom was absent (rating of N), but that other information and/or intra-interview cues implied that the symptom was present (rating of Y). The interviewer's assessment of "yes" would override the "no" response.

9. The follow-up sections on identity confusion and identity alteration are useful in making the interview flexible and individualized and in investigating the full severity spectrum of identity alteration. After the five sections (corresponding to the five symptoms) and the associated features section have been completed, the interviewer has the option of pursuing one or two of nine lines of questioning. These follow-up sections should be included if the interviewer suspects a Dissociative Disorder and believes that there may be identity disturbances whose scope needs to be explored further. If the interviewer does not have these suspicions, the follow-up sections need not be added.

   To decide which follow-up sections to go into, the interviewer simply "follows up" on the one or two most severe symptom areas that the subject mentioned in the interview, such as the use of different names to refer to himself or herself, the presence of internal dialogues, rapid mood changes, and feelings of possession. *No more than two follow-up sections need to be administered.* The questions in the follow-up sections inquire as to the personification and volition of internal entities or states of consciousness. These characteristics of symptoms indicate the extent of identity alteration and the presence of alter personalities. This is assessed by asking if, for example, the internal dialogues involve a consistent association with a visual image that has an age, name, or identity.

*10. Intra-interview dissociative cues that are suggestive of dissociative symptomatology are assessed at the end of the interview (see Questions 259–272). Fourteen behaviors or symptoms that may have been observed during the interview are rated. Each cue is operationally defined for clarity. The interviewer should be particularly familiar with (and vigilant for) these items, because no specific questions are asked. The interviewer uses his or her observations and judgment in rating these items, not the subject's responses.

*11. Following the interview, the interviewer should complete the Summary Score Sheet, which consists of two parts:

a. Rating of severity of five global symptoms associated with dissociative experiences: amnesia, depersonalization, derealization, identity confusion, and identity alteration. These ratings are recorded for all subjects, with or without a Dissociative Disorder. The Severity Rating Definitions should be used to rate these symptoms (see Chapter V).

b. Rating of presence or absence of a Dissociative Disorder and/or Acute Stress Disorder. If a Dissociative Disorder is present, the interviewer notes the specific disorder and records whether the subject has experienced a past episode or is currently manifesting the disorder (see Appendix 2).

Suggestions for a Shorter Interview

1. Questions indicated by an *asterisk* (*) are optional. They provide additional descriptive information. Because these items are not diagnostically discriminating for the Dissociative Disorders, overall diagnosis and scoring of the five symptom areas are not affected by the omission of these items. The interviewer can shorten the interview by skipping these questions.
2. Questions in *parentheses* are also optional, to be asked as needed to clarify the subject's responses. The interviewer can also add his or her questions in an attempt to follow up on a question and elicit sufficient information to rate it. Limiting these types of questions can also shorten the interview.
3. Questions that rule out drug or alcohol use or the presence of medical illness as etiological factors of dissociative symptoms may be skipped if the subject does not have a history of alcohol or drug use or medical illness (as reported in the Psychiatric History section).
4. The Psychiatric History section may be skipped if that information has been obtained previously.

IX. Interviewing Principles and Techniques

There are several interviewing techniques that should be followed to get the best results from the SCID-D. For experienced clinicians, many of these directives will be common sense. However, for those who have not had enough experience, the failure to use the following principles may make the difference between an informative session and an information-poor interview; between a spontaneous, animated interviewee and an inhibited, frightened subject; and between a satisfied interviewer and a frustrated interviewer. The principles espoused here are the result of extensive experience, including over 500 interviews conducted by five different interviewers in NIMH-funded field trials and in the multicenter field trials of the SCID-D (Steinberg et al. 1989–1993). Review of the interviewers' performance in administering these interviews and the training of SCID-D interviewers have contributed to what may be called "SCID-D wisdom."

It is hoped that the following principles are taken as reminders and reinforcers of abilities that are routinely kept in mind and continuously being developed. The use of these principles and techniques will enable the SCID-D to yield a psychologically rich interview, while being systematic and diagnostic. In addition, the SCID-D can be therapeutic by validating previously misdiagnosed cases of Dissociative Disorder. Although the interview is designed to gather information from the subject, the interviewer should consider equally both the structure of the interview and the state of mind of the subject. As it turns out, the most information-rich interviews are conducted by interviewers who allow the subject to feel comfortable to go into detailed descriptions.

1. *Invest time.* Administration of the SCID-D should be relaxed and should not be rushed. You will need to allow time for the subject to relay these multifaceted symptoms. However, do not spend too much time in the first section (Psychiatric History). The heart of the SCID-D is the five symptom areas, the associated features, and the follow-up sections. In fact, if you have already obtained a history, the first section may be skipped, and you can start with the first question in the Amnesia section. If necessary, the interview may also be shortened by skipping optional questions or follow-up sections.
2. *Guide the interview.* Let the subject know that you are competently guiding the course of the interview, that you will do your best to see that the interview goes smoothly, and that the subject may stop at any time, or may skip any question, if he or she wants to.
3. *Utilize follow-up questions.* Remember that the SCID-D is semistructured, so that the interviewer is free to follow up on a significant comment or anecdote. Some probing may be necessary, using questions that cannot be found explicitly in the interview. For example, if the subject, during a response to a depersonalization question, says, "I felt like I wasn't really there," the interviewer can ask the follow-up question, "Where did you feel you were?" Sometimes this type of follow-up leads to a more comprehensive description of the subject's symptom, or even a spontaneous elaboration regarding a different symptom. The subject may answer this question with "I was on a different planet" or "I felt like I was sleeping." More general follow-up questions include "What do you mean by that?" and "Can you say more?" which are useful in obtaining an elaboration on a response.
4. *Be tolerant of ambiguity.* Remember—it is more important for the subject to describe fully the vicissitudes of his or her dissociative experiences than for the interviewer to have the SCID-D questions answered "correctly." Diag-

nosis does not hinge on single responses. It is also okay for the subject to cross over into a discussion of other symptoms. Indeed, such spontaneous elaborations can be a clue to the existence of identity confusion and identity alteration.

5. *Practice active listening.* It is often useful to repeat or paraphrase a subject's response to convey a sense of understanding, to ensure a convergence of reference, and to keep the interview focused on dissociative symptoms.
6. *Do not confront the subject.* If a subject evades a question or does not answer a question adequately, it may be because he or she is distracted, feels apprehensive, does not understand the question, or is hearing voices telling him or her not to answer. A question that is misunderstood can be rephrased in a clearer way, perhaps with different words. Reference to the subject's evasiveness or misinterpretation is not suggested. The interviewer's responsibility is to make the subject feel as comfortable as possible.
7. *No need to apologize.* The interviewer need not say, "I know these questions seem unnecessary, but it's not much longer" or "I didn't write these questions, I'm only supposed to ask them." The interview may be a positive experience for the subject; it is often the first time he or she has been allowed to go into detail about dissociative experiences.
8. *Introducing seemingly similar questions.* The interview contains several questions about each symptom to address the multifaceted nature of dissociative symptoms. Some questions may be interpreted by the subject as redundant. In these cases, the interviewer has some options. If the new question covers additional aspects of a symptom that were already discussed, the interviewer can preface the question by stating, "You mentioned earlier that . . . ," and continue with the follow-up questions. If a question has been answered earlier, the interviewer has the option of skipping it or rephrasing it.

   Questions such as "How often did that occur?" can seem repetitive to the subject, especially if they are introduced each time they appear by a list of all options. I suggest that the interviewer, in general, *not* list all of the options in a frequency question. Instead, the interviewer may use his or her judgment in offering the most relevant choices, phrased in the form of a question. Often it is sufficient to say something like, "Would you say that that occurs monthly, weekly, or daily?" In addition, the "How often" questions can be skipped if you already know that the rating of the symptom in question is severe from previous frequency questions of that section.
9. *Do not overreact.* Do not get overly emotional in responding to the subject's experiences. A mild and consistent attitude of care and interest is best for the SCID-D interview.
10. *Make the interview a safe place.* If it seems as if the subject is anxious or apprehensive, you may ask whether he or she would like to take a break or to continue. Often, when asked, the subject may choose to continue. Make it clear that the subject is free to end the interview at any time. It is important to bear in mind that people with Dissociative Disorders may suffer ongoing anxiety or distress. Usually it is not the SCID-D questions that cause the anxiety.
11. *Do not press a tough question.* Skip a question if it appears difficult for the subject to answer (for whatever reason). Subjects with severe dissociative symptoms may spontaneously elaborate on trauma that occurred to them in their past. Lengthy responses should not be discouraged; however, care must be taken due to the sensitivity of the material. Similarly, subjects with Dissociative Identity Disorder (Multiple Personality Disorder) may change identity in the course of the interview. Interviewers should be prepared for the possibility of this occurrence.
12. *Allow the subject to elaborate.* These descriptions are essential for assessing the qualitative

nature of the subject's dissociative experiences. Each subject will manifest his or her symptoms in a different way—each subject has facets of symptoms that are unique to him or her. Often, a subject may describe a dissociative symptom that is different from the one asked about in a particular question. Such spontaneous elaboration is an important clue to a Dissociative Disorder, because the subject has revealed a close connection between his or her dissociative symptoms. Unlike individuals with bona fide Dissociative Disorders, malingerers and subjects who experience isolated symptoms due to organic disorders do not show such links between dissociative symptoms.

13. *Do not attempt to administer the interview to a patient who appears agitated or who does not want to cooperate.* This consideration is particularly relevant if you are assessing survivors of a group or community trauma or other individuals at risk for Acute Stress Disorder.

X. Diagnosis of the Dissociative Disorders

At this point in the rating of the interview, the symptom severity ratings have been completed. If the symptoms are severe enough to suggest the presence of a Dissociative Disorder, the interviewer is now ready to make a diagnosis. The SCID-D allows the clinician to move from a systematic assessment of symptoms to a systematic assessment of a Dissociative Disorder; however, the SCID-D does not permit the diagnosis of a specific nondissociative disorder.

How does one move from the symptom severity ratings to the diagnosis? The interviewer completes a summary of the severity ratings of the symptoms and evaluates this profile to decide which particular Dissociative Disorder is suggested by the constellation he or she has recorded.

The symptom profiles (Figure 2A) graphically illustrate the characteristic constellations of the five major Dissociative Disorders. The symptom profiles are a general summary and need not be adhered to rigidly. The same applies to the Diagnostic Work Sheets in Appendix 2. The seasoned interviewer's experience and judgment are the best basis for proceeding from symptom assessment to diagnosis, together with the information assembled in the severity rating sheets and the Diagnostic Work Sheets.

Diagnosis should always proceed from consideration of the core dissociative symptoms. The notation of moderate and severe dissociative symptoms on the Summary Score Sheet, as well as the interviewer's familiarity with DSM-IV criteria, should be used to determine whether a Dissociative Disorder is suggested. If the subject's symptoms were rated none to mild on all symptoms, a Dissociative Disorder may be ruled out. If, however, one or more symptoms was judged to be present at a high level of severity, the presence of a Dissociative Disorder should be considered. If the interviewer thinks that a Dissociative Disorder is not present, he or she checks the box for "no evidence of Dissociative Disorder." On the other hand, if the subject's symptomatology supports DSM-IV criteria for a Dissociative Disorder, the interviewer marks the box for "meets criteria for a Dissociative Disorder."

To achieve a diagnostic assessment, it is important to remember that diagnosis does not hinge on the subject's answer to any single question on the SCID-D. A positive response regarding one dissociative symptom often has several possible ramifications, which must be explored through persistence with related questions. Isolated dissociative symptoms may occur in a number of different psychiatric syndromes, both dissociative and nondissociative. An isolated dissociative symptom, such as use of an alternate name or an amnestic episode, is insufficient grounds for diagnosis. To provide evidence sufficient for an accurate diagnosis, the symptom must exist in combination with other symptoms that, as a group, conform to the characteristic pattern of one of the five disorders outlined in the Diagnostic Work Sheets in Appendix 2.

If it is believed that a diagnosis of a Dissociative Disorder is appropriate, the interviewer should then examine the pattern of symptoms and symptom severity to decide which Dissociative Disorder is suggested. For this process, the interviewer should compare the overall pattern of symptoms reported with the constellations of symptoms enumerated in the Diagnostic Work Sheets (in support of the more global DSM-IV criteria) for the various Dissociative Disorders. These resources should be used to assess the correspondence between the symptoms and the DSM-IV criteria for the Dissociative Disorders.

For uncertain cases in which it is not clear which disorder the symptom constellation most closely resembles, the interviewer may find guidance in the final section of this chapter, "Distinguishing Among the Dissociative Disorders." Keep in mind that difficulty in assessing the exact type of Dissociative Disorder in individuals with severe dissociative symptoms may indicate (but not necessarily so) the presence of Dissociative Disorder Not Otherwise Specified. Moreover, as Cases 2 and 3 in Chapter XIV indicate, some patients who are diagnosed on 6-month follow-up as having Dissociative Identity Disorder may present initially with Dissociative Disorder Not Otherwise Specified due to inadequate symptom disclosure during the initial SCID-D interview. Alternatively, diagnostic uncertainty may indicate insufficient familiarity or sensitivity on the interviewer's part with dissociative psychopathology, or perhaps a subject who is not yet fully comfortable with disclosing his or her symptoms. In the latter case, an additional SCID-D interview should be performed at a later date so that the subject may feel more comfortable with the interviewer and with the SCID-D. In many cases, subjects with Dissociative Disorders have been misdiagnosed for many years and do not understand their dissociative experiences or may have come to understand their symptoms erroneously under a different pathological description. Multiple interviews may be required for these subjects to verbalize their symptoms and to express themselves accurately.

The interviewer should not adhere to the symptom profiles in a restrictive fashion, because each person with a Dissociative Disorder will manifest differences in symptomatology. For example, in Dissociative Identity Disorder (Multiple Personality Disorder), identity confusion may be low for subjects who have high interpersonality amnesia (i.e., each personality does not get feedback from or about the other personalities and is not confused about his or her identity). In these patients, identity alteration is usually high.

As the interviewer increases his or her familiarity with the SCID-D and with individuals who have dissociative and nondissociative disorders, he or she may be able to bypass the Diagnostic Work Sheets. However, the Summary Score Sheet should always be used, for the patient's record.

The Diagnostic Work Sheets, like the Severity Rating Definitions, are to be used as general guidelines. In this case, they enable the interviewer to use responses to SCID-D questions to verify the satisfaction of DSM-IV criteria for a given Dissociative Disorder. How does the interviewer know if the DSM-IV criteria are satisfied? The SCID-D operationalizes the DSM-IV definitions by stating intermediate diagnostic criteria that support the respective DSM-IV criteria. For example, DSM-IV Dissociative Identity Disorder Criterion A of the Diagnostic Work Sheet requires

> the existence within the individual of two or more distinct personalities or personality states (each with its own relatively enduring pattern of perceiving, relating to, and thinking about the environment and one's self).

This DSM-IV criterion is followed by five SCID-D criteria, each of which is further broken down into items that correspond to specific SCID-D responses. The SCID-D criteria operationalize the DSM-IV criteria by incorporating specific experiences and behaviors suggestive of Dissociative Identity Disorder—for example, SCID-D Criterion 2:

> Persistent feeling that two or more people exist within themselves, as indicated by at least one of the following: a) persistent feeling that they are two different people, one going through the motions of life and the other observing (refer to SCID-D items #81, #82); b) persistent feeling that they act as if they were a different person or they are told by others that they seem like a different person (SCID-D items #34, #34a); and c) use of different names, or being called by others by different names (not nicknames or an alias used only to facilitate illegal activity). (SCID-D items #87, #88)

After a given Diagnostic Work Sheet has been completed, there are exclusionary criteria that check for the existence of symptoms or disorders that will rule out the existence of the Dissociative Disorder in question. If the subject's symptoms do not meet the criteria for a given Dissociative Disorder based on the results of that specific Diagnostic Work Sheet, the interviewer may refer back to the symptom profiles and explore the possibility of a different diagnosis.

Finally, when a diagnosis has been made, the interviewer fills out the appropriate box on the Summary Score Sheet. The Summary Score Sheet should now contain 1) severity ratings for all five symptoms, 2) an indication of the presence or absence of a Dissociative Disorder and/or Acute Stress Disorder, and 3) the specific Dissociative Disorder diagnosis.

Distinguishing Among the Dissociative Disorders

The Dissociative Disorders are classified together because all involve a predominant "disruption in the usually integrative functions of consciousness, memory, identity, or perception of the environment" (DSM-IV, p. 490). The Dissociative Disorders differ, however, in their symptom profiles—that is, in the presence and severity of particular dissociative symptoms. Differential diagnosis is a matter of assessing a patient's dissociative symptoms in terms of the characteristic symptom constellations of each disorder.

To distinguish among the disorders, each symptom should be evaluated by considering context, content, course, and predisposing factors. For example, take amnesia:

In Dissociative Amnesia, amnesia is the predominant disturbance. The amnesia occurs as a single acute episode and follows a particular psychosocial stress.

In Dissociative Fugue, amnesia is not the sole disturbance, and it occurs in conjunction with wandering from home and alteration in identity. The amnesia is generalized and may cover the period during which an alteration in identity occurred. As with Dissociative Amnesia, onset and termination are abrupt, and the amnesia occurs as a single acute episode. The fugue usually begins following severe psychosocial stress.

In Depersonalization Disorder, amnesia is not a clinically significant symptom. In Dissociative Disorder Not Otherwise Specified, amnesia typically occurs in connection with an alteration in identity. The amnesia may be chronic and recurrent.

In Dissociative Identity Disorder (Multiple Personality Disorder), amnesia occurs in conjunction with depersonalization, derealization, identity confusion, and alteration in identity. The amnesia varies and may be circumscribed, continuous, or generalized. It is chronic and recurrent. The amnesia develops during the course of an illness that in nearly all cases is preceded by a long history of physical, emotional, and/or sexual abuse during childhood.

Finally, in Acute Stress Disorder, amnesia occurs in conjunction with depersonalization and derealization but without significant identity confusion and alteration. In addition, the symptoms of Acute Stress Disorder last for a minimum of 2 days and a maximum of 4 weeks; their onset is within 4 weeks of a traumatic event that involves the person as a participant or witness.

In summary, an isolated dissociative symptom may occur in several of the five Dissociative Disorders as well as in Acute Stress Disorder. However, rather than looking only at a single symptom, the diagnostician must evaluate the symptom for characteristic distinguishing features and the presence of the entire constellation of symptoms that typifies a specific disorder. The other four symptoms will also manifest differently in the different disorders. Knowledge of these differential manifestations is helpful in recognizing a particular Dissociative Disorder when the interviewer is confronted with an assortment of symptoms. Initial hunches may then be followed up with systematic assessment of all the symptoms, as is done in the SCID-D.

XI. Overlapping Symptoms Among Dissociative and Nondissociative Disorders

Dissociative Disorders and nondissociative disorders may display overlapping symptoms. This section reviews the distinguishing features of overlapping symptoms in Dissociative Disorders and nondissociative disorders. Specific features of the isolated symptom are described within the context of each syndrome in which the symptom might occur.

Auditory hallucinations and identity disturbances, for example, may occur in several quite different disorders. This overlap can produce misinterpretation or confusion, which is remedied when the symptoms are examined for distinguishing traits. Analyzing potentially overlapping symptoms helps in differential diagnosis by 1) placing the symptom in relation to any other symptoms that are present, 2) examining the content of the symptom, 3) examining the severity and duration of the symptom, and 4) examining the course of the symptom and of the illness in which it exists.

The overlap of hallucinations and identity disturbance between Dissociative Disorders and other disorders frequently leads to misinterpretation and may result in misdiagnosis. For example, a patient who has Dissociative Identity Disorder (Multiple Personality Disorder) and describes auditory hallucinations is likely to be diagnosed as having a Psychotic Disorder by clinicians unfamiliar with dissociative symptoms and Dissociative Disorders. Such a clinician may fail to distinguish between auditory hallucinations that derive from coherent alter personalities and those that derive from a chaotic, psychotic episode. Similarly, a patient who has Schizophrenia may exhibit identity disturbances that seem superficially similar to identity alteration in Dissociative Identity Disorder. However, a clinician who can distinguish between the primitive, delusional identity disturbance of Schizophrenia and the complex, coherent identity disturbance of Dissociative Identity Disorder will be able to make an accurate diagnosis.

There are several potentially overlapping symptoms other than auditory hallucinations or identity disturbances. Schneiderian symptoms may be seen in Schizophrenia, Dissociative Identity Disorder, Bipolar Disorder, and other disorders. The symptom of depersonalization may occur in patients with many syndromes, as well as in some control subjects. In the case of depersonalization, the isolated symptom would be checked for 1) a relationship to other dissociative and nondissociative symptoms, 2) content or nature of the depersonalization, 3) SCID-D severity rating, and 4) the history of the depersonalization and the course of the syndrome. If appropriate, the diagnosis of Depersonalization Disorder would then be evaluated. Symptoms of derealization or amnesia would be assessed in the same way. We will consider individuals with four psychological conditions: Dissociative Identity Disorder, Schizophrenia, Major Depression, and no psychiatric illness.

How are auditory hallucinations present in Dissociative Identity Disorder? Internal dialogues in Dissociative Identity Disorder occur in the context of other dissociative symptoms. The voices represent internal personalities talking among themselves. The voices are usually thought to derive from inside the patient's head (occasionally they are perceived as coming from the outside). The voice is associated with consistent age, talents, and attitudes and occasionally takes control of the body. Signs of the symptom are intermittent.

Auditory hallucinations in patients with Schizophrenia manifest differently. Voices occur exclusively during the course of a psychotic disturbance. This is surmised by the presence of psychotic symptoms such as delusions, impaired reality testing, and loose associations. The voices are part of a general bizarre ideation that often involves external individuals (not internal personalities). The hallucinations are typically perceived as arising from outside the person's head. Functioning is markedly low in the schizophrenic patient, and the illness is continuous for at least 6 months. The course of Schizophrenia is downward; early levels of higher functioning are normally not regained.

In Major Depression, internal voices occur in the context of the depression, involving themes of inadequacy, guilt, or death. The voices are described as being "inner voices," arising from inside the person's head.

In individuals without psychiatric illness, internal dialogues occur in the context of thinking, remembering, or planning. These dialogues are perceived as inside the head and are more like thoughts than real voices.

Identity disturbance also differs in each of these psychological conditions. Identity disturbance in Dissociative Identity Disorder occurs in the context of a dissociative syndrome. This is true if the confusion or alteration is accompanied by amnesia, depersonalization, or derealization. In Dissociative Identity Disorder, the identity disturbance is the predominant disturbance. The identity disturbance involves recurrent or persistent alterations in identity. Level of functioning within the population of Dissociative Identity Disorder patients varies, with any impairment usually being temporary.

In Schizophrenia, the identity disturbance is somewhat different. The disturbance occurs in the context of loose associations, flat affect, and psychotic delusions. The sense of self is impaired (loss of ego boundaries). Identity disturbance is usually not the predominant disturbance. Identity alterations typically involve supernatural beings or fictional or famous people and are often associated with delusional identifications with these people.

In Major Depression, individuals have a low sense of self-esteem and often have conflict about their lives. However, the depression is the predominant disturbance, and identity alteration does not occur.

In subjects without psychiatric illness, identity problems involve mild identity conflicts, common among adolescents and in "mid-life crises." These occurrences are typically transient and normally do not involve dysfunction. Changing roles is a mild, nonpathological form of identity alteration, which is typically not associated with dysfunction in any way.

In summary, an isolated symptom may be seen in many quite different syndromes. However, diagnosis should never hinge on the presence of a single symptom. Diagnosis requires an evaluation of the symptom for the presence of characteristic distinguishing features along with the presence of the entire constellation of symptoms typical of the disorder.

The Dissociative Disorders may coexist with a variety of other psychiatric disorders. Several points should be considered in evaluating whether there is a coexisting disorder:

- Dissociative Disorders may coexist with alcohol use, drug use, and organic disorders (i.e., temporal lobe epilepsy), but only if the dissociative symptoms are not induced by these factors solely.
- In Dissociative Identity Disorder, one or more personalities may have a particular symptom or disorder that the other personalities do not share. For example, one of the personalities may suffer from Major Depression.
- Because the Dissociative Disorders are all Axis I disorders, they may coexist with the Personality Disorders (Axis II). For example, Depersonalization Disorder or Dissociative Identity Disorder may coexist with Borderline Personality Disorder.
- A Dissociative Disorder cannot coexist with a psychotic disorder, such as Schizophrenia. However, a person with a Dissociative Disorder may appear to have a transient psychotic episode, often due to age regression and/or flash-

backs to traumatic events. Dissociative Identity Disorder is particularly likely to be misdiagnosed as Schizophrenia because of the characteristic auditory (and sometimes visual) hallucinations that occur in Dissociative Identity Disorder.

- Depersonalization Disorder is diagnosed if the depersonalization is the primary symptom and if the predominant disturbance is of a dissociative nature. However, depersonalization is often masked by symptoms of anxiety, panic, and/or depression; a thorough investigation of dissociative symptomatology is necessary for correct differential diagnosis.

SCID-D Symptom Profiles in Psychiatric Patients and Nonpsychiatric Control Subjects (Figure 3)

The presence and severity of dissociative symptomatology varies considerably across different groups. People with Dissociative Disorders, of course, experience the most severe dissociative symptoms, and within the Dissociative Disorders, people with Dissociative Identity Disorder manifest the most severe symptoms. People with *non*dissociative disorders have also been found to experience dissociative symptoms. Some disorders have been found to include a great deal of dissociative symptomatology.

FIGURE 3. SCID-D symptom profiles in psychiatric patients and nonpsychiatric control subjects.
Source. Data from Steinberg M, Rounsaville B, Cicchetti D: "The Structured Clinical Interview for DSM-III-R Dissociative Disorders: Preliminary Report on a New Diagnostic Instrument." *American Journal of Psychiatry* 147:76–82, 1990.

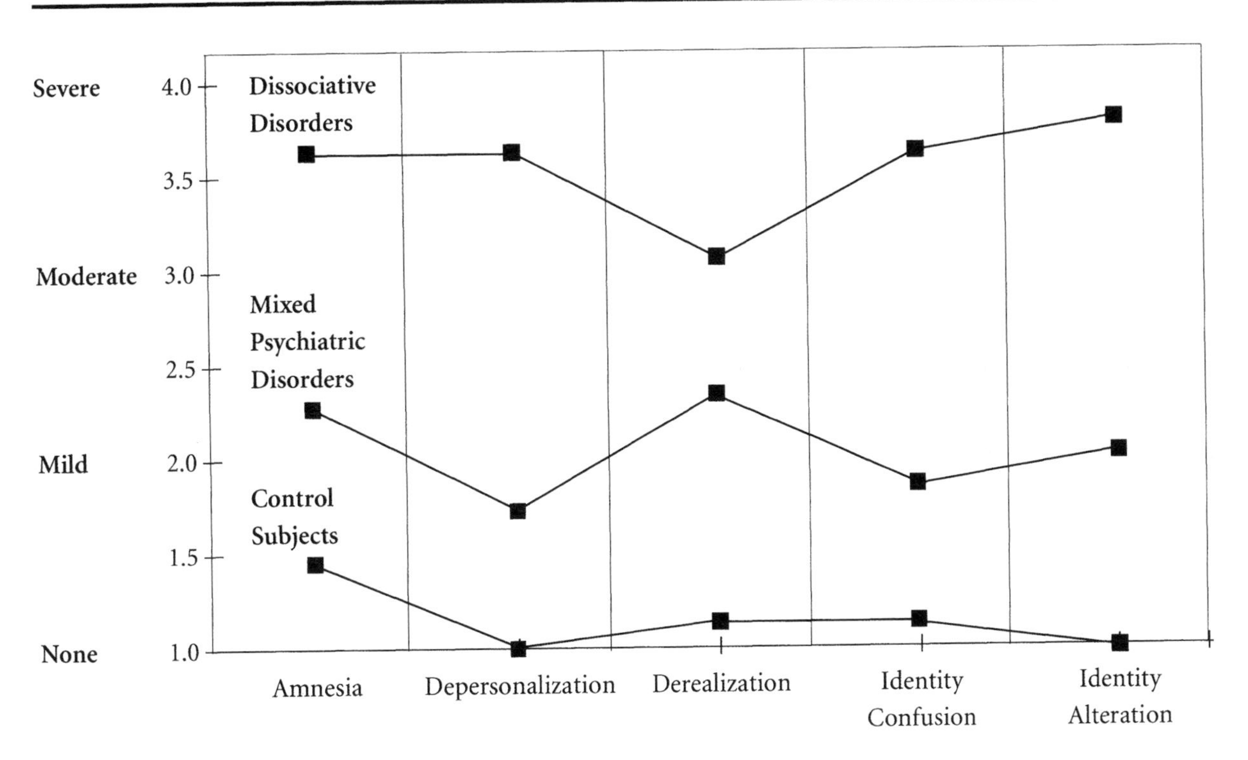

These include Posttraumatic Stress Disorder (Spiegel 1988; Spiegel and Cardeña 1990) and Anorexia (Goodwin and Attias 1993; Torem 1986). Additionally, Borderline Personality Disorder has been described as involving moderate amounts of dissociative symptomatology (Boon and Draijer 1991; Dinges 1977). Subjects without psychiatric illness report mild, nonpathological dissociative symptomatology, and psychiatric patients with a variety of psychiatric disorders manifest mild to moderate dissociative symptomatology (Steinberg et al. 1990).

Figure 3 is a graph of the symptom profiles of Dissociative Disorder patients, mixed psychiatric patients, and control subjects. Control subjects tend to score between none and mild (1–2) for all five symptoms. Mixed psychiatric patients score between none and moderate (1–3). People with Dissociative Disorders score between moderate and severe (3–4). As mentioned, patients with Dissociative Identity Disorder typically score within a range of 17–20 for all the symptoms, with points normally plotted at 3 or 4 (moderate to severe) for each symptom.

Review of Symptoms in the Context of Schizophrenia and Dissociative Identity Disorder (Table 7)

Table 7 demonstrates that although there may be overlapping symptoms in Dissociative Identity Disorder and Schizophrenia, there are also distinguishing features. *Column 1* lists symptoms characteristic of Schizophrenia; *Column 2* identifies symptoms that may occur in either disorder; *Column 3* consists of symptoms characteristic of Dissociative Identity Disorder. Differentiation of overlapping symptoms depends on 1) examining the symptom in relation to any other symptoms that are present; 2) examining the content of the symptom; 3) examining the severity of the symptom, including dysfunction and/or distress; and 4) examining the course of the symptom and of the illness in which it exists.

TABLE 7. Review of symptoms in the context of Schizophrenia and Dissociative Identity Disorder (DID) (Multiple Personality Disorder)

Symptoms characteristic of Schizophrenia	Overlapping symptoms potentially present in both Schizophrenia and DID	Symptoms characteristic of DID
Usually isolated symptoms (none to mild severity ratings on the SCID-D). Symptoms occur in the context of bizarre delusions or other psychotic symptoms.	Dissociative symptoms	Recurrent to persistent dissociative symptoms (moderate to severe severity ratings on the SCID-D).
Lack of sense of identity and one's role in society.	Identity confusion/disturbance	Recurrent and consistent alterations in one's identity.
Hallucinations other than the voices of alter personalities. These are perceived as occurring primarily outside the patient's head.	Auditory hallucinations and internal dialogues	Auditory hallucinations reflect dialogues between alter personalities. These voices are perceived as occurring inside the patient's head. Often described as similar to thoughts.
Bizarre delusions, paranoid delusions, and any other delusions that do not involve the other personalities, e.g., "The CIA is out to get me."	Schneiderian symptoms and delusions	Only delusions are "delusions of several personalities" or of other bodily changes representative of the different personalities.
Thinking characterized by incoherence or marked loosening of associations.	Other psychotic symptoms	Absent in DID.
Catatonic behavior.		Absent in DID.
Chronic flat affect.		Absent in DID.
Impaired reality testing.	Reality testing	Intact reality testing; "as if" descriptions of dissociative symptoms are typical.
"If mood episodes have occurred during active-phase symptoms, their total duration has been brief relative to the duration of the active and residual periods" (DSM-IV, pp. 285–286).	Comorbid diagnoses	The full depressive or manic syndrome may coexist with the dissociative syndrome.
"One or more areas of functioning such as work, interpersonal relations, or self-care are markedly below the level achieved prior to the onset" (DSM-IV, p. 285).	Impairment in functioning	Any impairment in functioning is usually temporary, with eventual full return to premorbid level of functioning.
"Continuous signs of the disturbance for at least 6 months" (DSM-IV, p. 285).	Course of symptoms and syndrome	Signs of the disturbance may be intermittent. Rapid fluctuations in symptoms, mood, and degree of impairment may occur.

XII. Feedback and Follow-Up Interviews

The SCID-D is not only effective in diagnosis and assessment but also in treatment planning. SCID-D research has indicated that many patients both welcome and benefit from an opportunity for feedback after the interview. In many cases, a brief feedback period immediately following administration of the instrument may be sufficient. After the interview, the subject should be thanked for participating. If the subject did not report significant dissociative symptoms, the interviewer can point out that the SCID-D was designed to assess certain types of symptoms that are not routinely talked about and that are often associated with stressful and/or traumatic events. With subjects who reported a significant level of dissociative symptomatology, information about dissociation should be conveyed to them in their own words.

In some instances, the clinician may want to consider scheduling a longer feedback interview for the patient. Patients diagnosed with Dissociative Identity Disorder (Multiple Personality Disorder) or Dissociative Disorder Not Otherwise Specified may benefit from more detailed explanations of their disorders, particularly if their symptoms have caused severe distress or dysfunction, or they may have a number of questions about their family history or present treatment regimen.

Feedback interviews have been helpful to SCID-D subjects for a number of reasons. In some cases, feedback assists the patient in moving forward in his or her present therapy. One subject in the SCID-D field study reported that the instrument provided "a springboard" for subsequent therapy sessions and felt that he now had "a handle on the real problem." For other patients, feedback interviews provide them with a new perspective on their family of origin or allow them to begin their emotional recovery. Case 4 in Part III includes a summary of a patient's feedback interview. The young woman in this case study had used the time interval between administration of the SCID-D and the feedback interview to reflect on the symptomatic behaviors of other family members and to participate more assertively in her therapy. Thus, feedback interviews may have a therapeutic dimension in their own right, as well as providing patient education.

Due to previous lack of systematic assessment of dissociative symptoms, many subjects experience the SCID-D as their first opportunity to describe their symptoms in their own words to a receptive listener. Some persons come to the interview with the fear that their dissociative episodes mark them as "crazy" or psychotic. It is essential that the interviewer provide reassurance that dissociative symptoms do not suggest the presence of psychosis. If the subject's symptoms are severe, or if he or she appears to have a Dissociative Disorder, you should discuss the reality and importance of their symptoms, as well as the relationship between trauma and dissociation. For example, you might tell the subject that his or her experiences are very significant, deserve to be taken seriously, and are more common than people ordinarily think. It is not unusual for subjects diagnosed with a Dissociative Disorder on the SCID-D to be surprised at having their symptoms validated by a clinician who understands the nature of their disorder. If a referral is indicated, recommend that the patient consult an experienced therapist who understands the nature and significance of dissociation. If the subject has been previously misdiagnosed, emphasize that dissociative symptoms are elusive and require specific strategies and diagnostic tools for accurate assessment.

In addition, discuss the dissociation in an "adaptive" manner—that is, as a defense mechanism that enabled them to adapt to some very difficult or painful past experiences and that is still operating in the present because of these painful occurrences. Many people with Dissociative Disorders are very creative and used their creative capacities to help them cope with childhood trauma. Last, you should observe that Dissociative Disorders have a high rate of responsiveness to therapy and that with proper treatment, their prognosis is quite good.

Follow-Up Interviews

Although most patients will not require a second administration of the SCID-D, the instrument's good-to-excellent interrater reliability makes it an effective diagnostic tool in cases necessitating a 6-month follow-up. These fall into four major categories: 1) a subset of patients with Dissociative Disorder Not Otherwise Specified (DDNOS), 2) patients presenting with global or severe amnesia, 3) patients with Acute Stress Disorder, and 4) some forensic cases.

The first category includes patients who are initially diagnosed as having DDNOS whose symptoms were not fully disclosed. On 6-month follow-up, further disclosure indicates that a subset of these patients meet the full criteria for Dissociative Identity Disorder (Multiple Personality Disorder).

Patients in the second category—with severe or global amnesia—frequently require follow-up because the amnesia may prevent sufficient symptom disclosure during the first interview to permit accurate differential diagnosis.

The third group—patients diagnosed with Acute Stress Disorder— should receive a 6-month follow-up to evaluate the presence of ongoing symptoms and/or to rule out the possibility of an underlying Dissociative Disorder.

The fourth group includes subjects involved in civil or criminal cases, who may need to be evaluated more than once because of the adversarial nature of legal proceedings or a change of venue.

In addition to these subcategories, clinicians and researchers may find follow-up administrations of the SCID-D helpful in monitoring a patient's symptom severity or general progress in therapy.

XIII. Use of the SCID-D in Research

Although this *Interviewer's Guide* was compiled primarily for use by clinicians, the SCID-D is also a tool with many applications in a number of different areas of research. To begin with psychiatry itself, over 500 SCID-D interviews have been administered to date in investigations of dissociative symptoms in patients with a variety of psychiatric disorders, ranging from eating disorders (Boon and Draijer 1991) to obsessive-compulsive disorder (Goff et al. 1991, 1992) to schizophrenia (Steinberg 1995). Case studies have been presented by Hall and Steinberg (1993) and in this *Interviewer's Guide.*

In addition, given DSM-IV's introduction of two new categories—Dissociative Trance Disorder (as a subtype of Dissociative Disorder Not Otherwise Specified) and Acute Stress Disorder—the SCID-D can be used in research investigations of these syndromes. Areas for further research include the phenomenology of these disorders, as well as possible refinement of present DSM-IV criteria and classifications.

Additional possibilities for research include the sociology of medicine, including cross-cultural studies, epidemiology (longitudinal and multigenerational studies), comparison of dissociative symptomatology in dissociative and nondissociative disorders, qualitative studies of dissociation, and outcome studies, including pharmacological treatments of dissociation. At present, no controlled double-blind studies have been done that compare the relative efficacies of pharmacotherapy and psychotherapy or the relative efficacies of different models of psychotherapy for Dissociative Disorders.

With regard to pharmacology in particular, it is highly likely that a variety of agents will prove to be effective in the treatment of depersonalization and other dissociative symptoms. The SCID-D is an instrument that facilitates medication trials, in that its Summary Score Sheet can be used to record the severity as well as the presence of dissociative symptoms. This record would establish subjects' baselines prior to the medication trials, and thereby allow for the matching of subject groups for comparative studies.

The specific features of the SCID-D that recommend it as an instrument in research include 1) its systematic assessment of the presence of dissociative symptoms and disorders, 2) its ability to quantify symptomatology in terms of the severity of each symptom, 3) its comprehensive evaluation of the many dimensions (including nonverbal dimensions) of the subject's endorsed experiences, and 4) its good-to-excellent interrater reliability. The SCID-D offers the clinician-researcher a means for collecting quantitatively ample and qualitatively rich data. The Severity Rating Definitions allow researchers to compare the results of studies at different sites on the basis of a common scale. Quantitative data can also be easily used in data processing.

PART III

CASE STUDIES

XIV. Four Sample Case Studies

This section of the *Interviewer's Guide* contains four sample case studies, arranged as follows:

- A sample case study, "The Inner Sanctum," in which the reader is invited to follow a trained SCID-D interviewer through the process of differential diagnosis of a Dissociative Disorder using DSM-IV criteria. Figure 4, "SCID-D Decision Tree for the Dissociative Disorders," is included in Appendix 1 as a visual summary of the verbal descriptions and explanations in Case 1.
- Two case studies, "The Angry Genie in the Bottle" and "The Man Without A Past," are presented in the form of psychological reports. You may find these case studies helpful in learning how to use the SCID-D in writing psychological evaluations. These evaluations can be included in patient charts for symptom documentation, as well as in patient education and treatment planning.
- A concluding full-length case history, "The Postman Rings Twice," provides a detailed example of a SCID-D interview with a patient with coexisting seizure disorder. Although the patient in this full-length study was in no way involved with the criminal justice system, we have included an additional decision tree ("Differential Diagnosis of Dissociative Symptoms") in Appendix 1 to illustrate the clinical and evidentiary applications of the SCID-D in forensic evaluations.

These particular case studies were selected for the *Interviewer's Guide* as instructive instances of the range of the SCID-D's clinical applications and the interview's ability to detect previously undiagnosed dissociative disturbances in a wide cross-section of the psychiatric population. The four individuals whose cases are summarized here represent very different ethnic and educational backgrounds, presenting complaints, comorbid disorders, and differential diagnoses. All four exemplify the clinical applications of the SCID-D in diagnostic assessments, patient education, and treatment planning. In all cases, identifying details regarding age, occupation, ethnic background, geographic location, and the like have been changed to protect confidentiality.

This concluding chapter of the *Interviewer's Guide* is followed by an appendix that reproduces the "Depersonalization" segment of the SCID-D interview, allowing the reader to observe an experienced interviewer's notations and scoring.

Case 1: The Inner Sanctum

Case 1, the practice exercise, concerns a patient who describes her dissociative symptoms as "going inside"—retreating into her private world. Ms. S. is a 36-year-old divorced white woman currently living with her boyfriend and two children. She is currently employed as a financial analyst and has held her present position for 4 years. She has been in outpatient therapy with her current therapist for the past 5 years. Ms. S. has not been previously hospitalized for psychiatric reasons.

The report that follows is a summary of her responses in the five symptom areas, together with excerpts from her interviews, to allow assessment of the severity of her symptoms. You may want to refer to the Severity Rating Definitions on pp. 18–22 in the course of this practice exercise. The interviewer compares Ms. S.'s responses with DSM-IV criteria for syndromes that are characterized by the predominance of each specific dissociative symptom. The interviewer reviews the symptoms, decides whether the diagnosis of a Dissociative Disorder is warranted, and then decides which Dissociative Disorder will be considered in the differential diagnosis. The next step requires comparisons of this patient's symptom profile with those that are characteristic of the five Dissociative Disorders. Knowledge of exclusionary factors and the subsumptive hierarchy of Dissociative Disorders must be applied throughout the process. Dissociative Identity Disorder, being the most severe syndrome, will subsume any other Dissociative Disorder diagnosis. The Diagnostic Work Sheets can be used as guides during the differential diagnosis. You may also find it helpful to track the course of the differential diagnosis on Figure 4 (p. 91) and Figure 6 (p. 93) in Appendix 1.

Assessment of the Five Dissociative Symptoms

1. Amnesia. Ms. S. reports experiencing large gaps in her memory: "A month would go by that I couldn't account for." Her replies to Question 4 and the interviewer's spontaneous follow-up question indicate that her amnesia is extensive in terms of the aspects of her life that it affects and occurs frequently. In addition, this transcript excerpt illustrates the interviewer's use of appropriate probing follow-up questions, as well as the subject's volunteering of sufficient detail to aid the interviewer's assessment.

Interviewer: Have you ever felt as if there were large gaps in your memory?

Patient: Yes. Um, it'll be days, a couple of days; it usually never lasts for more than a couple of days, where I won't be able to remember what happened.

Interviewer: Can you describe what you mean by that?

Patient: It will seem to me that it's still a Friday, and then I'll realize that it's Monday and I'll search my memory to figure out what happened over the weekend.

Interviewer: So it feels as if from the Friday to the Monday, you have gaps for that time.

Patient: It's like if you've ever driven in the car and you're driving along, and you know where you're supposed to go, um, and all of a sudden you're there, but you can't remember how you got there.

Interviewer: How often would you say that experience occurs?

Patient: I try to forget it. I don't concentrate on how often it happens. Sometimes it will happen a lot and then other times I'll go for a long time and it won't happen at all.

Interviewer: What makes you aware that time passed and you weren't able to remember what you did during that time?

Patient: Um *[pauses]* all of a sudden I'll be standing someplace. It happened to me recently, so I'm thinking of standing at the sink. I all of a sudden realized I was standing at the sink, and I thought, "What time is it?" and I looked at the time; and then I go through a process of figuring out what time it is, what day it is, and then I start thinking [about] what happened. So I just all of a sudden find myself someplace.

The same features characterize Ms. S.'s exchanges with the interviewer for two subsequent amnesia items (Questions 6 and 7). The interviewer notes intra-interview amnesia, as well as Ms. S.'s lengthy pauses during her descriptions of amnesia, suggestive of significant emotional responses to SCID-D questions:

Interviewer: Have you ever had a time in which you had difficulty remembering your daily activities?

Patient: Yeah.

Interviewer: Can you describe what that is like or what you forgot?

Patient: Oh, I forgot some dentist appointments, doctors' appointments. I'll forget clothes in the dryer. I'll forget, *[pauses]* I'll thought I have made the bed and then I'll realize that, I'll go in and I'll see that I haven't made the bed. I will be sure that I've done something and then I'll—is that what you mean?

Interviewer: Yes. Have you ever found yourself in a place and been unable to remember how or why you went there?
Patient: Yes.
Interviewer: Where did you find yourself?
Patient: Um, found myself in the therapist's office, not knowing how or why I got there. I found myself in the grocery store. I found myself at the movies. Yes.

Ms. S. also endorsed episodes of "coming to" in the downtown area of the city where she lives and not remembering where she had parked her car. When asked whether she has ever had difficulty remembering personal information (Question 15), she recalled going to a job interview and finding herself unable to remember her age, telephone number, or home address. These amnestic episodes have occurred without the use of drugs or alcohol and in the absence of acute medical illness.

Amnesia Severity Rating—Severe. Due to the *nature* of Ms. S.'s amnesia (difficulty remembering basic personal information and daily activities) and high *frequency* (daily or weekly gaps in her memory), her amnesia is rated as severe. (See Severity Rating Definitions for further information.)

2. **Depersonalization.** Ms. S. endorses several different manifestations of depersonalization. In response to Questions 40, 41, 46, and 47, she supplies some details of her feelings of detachment and inner splitting:

Interviewer: Have you ever felt like a stranger to yourself?
Patient: Yes.
Interviewer: What is that experience like?
Patient: Well, I never have a real sense of who I am or what I like, or, um, if I'm ever really sure about anything.
Interviewer: How often do you have that feeling?
Patient: I think, a lot. There probably isn't a day that goes by that I don't have a sense of that in some interaction.
Interviewer: Have you ever felt as if a part of your body or your whole being was foreign to you?
Patient: I have a feeling like there is part of me and there are parts of me that give me the creeps, and that makes me sick to my stomach . . .
Interviewer: Have you ever felt that you were going through the motions of life, but you really felt detached from your behavior or that you were living in a dream?
Patient: Yes. Yes, I will see myself going through motions sometimes and think, "Why can't I feel this?"; am I . . . it's almost a sense of my body's just moving and I'm not really there, that type [of] thing.
Interviewer: Have you ever felt as if you were two different people, one going through the motions of life and the other part observing?
Patient: Yeah.
Interviewer: What's that like?
Patient: Well, that's a feeling of going inside. It's that feeling of going inside.

In addition to supplying the interviewer with numerous examples of depersonalization (feeling like a stranger to herself, feeling detached from parts of her body, feeling detached from her behavior, and feeling divided between an observing and participating self), Ms. S. indicates a high level of distress connected with this symptom. Her remark that she sometimes feels nauseated appears to reflect distress in somatic form.

At another point during this section of the SCID-D, she remarks that these episodes "make me feel depressed." Also in this section of the interview, she reports that her behavior and emotions are not always in her control: she has occasionally found herself in a bar, flirting with a stranger, and has found herself crying uncontrollably and sucking her thumb for reasons that she cannot explain. She describes these episodes as "frightening" and adds that they occur weekly. These descriptions provide the interviewer with further evidence that Ms. S. suffers from identity alteration, because of her reference to other "parts" of herself that upset her, and because of the age regression suggested by the thumb sucking.

Depersonalization Severity Rating—Severe. Ms. S.'s depersonalization is rated as severe due to the recurrent nature of this symptom. In addition, the nature of her symptom—specifically, depersonalization that has interfered with her ability to function and has lasted for several days at least—is qualitatively of a severe nature. (See Severity Rating Definitions for further information.)

3. Derealization. Ms. S. has experienced derealization episodes in which familiar surroundings and people feel unreal or unfamiliar. Her discomfort with these experiences manifests in her lengthy pauses during her answers. Once again, she uses the phrase "going inside" to describe her reaction to these uncomfortable feelings:

Interviewer: Have you ever felt as if familiar surroundings or people you knew seemed unfamiliar or unreal?
Patient: *[pauses for 10 seconds]* Yeah, I have a sense of that. When that feeling comes, it only lasts a split second and then I'm inside.
Interviewer: Then you retreat inside?
Patient: Yeah.

Ms. S. also mentions a sense of confusion about the reality of her surroundings, in reply to Question 84. Note that Ms. S.'s answer indicates that her confusion has a temporal as well as a spatial dimension:

Interviewer: Have you ever felt puzzled as to what's real and what's unreal in your surroundings?
Patient: *[pauses]* Yeah, I guess I have.
Interviewer: What kinds of things would be puzzling?
Patient: *[pauses]* The bathroom or the living room. They'll seem unreal. I'll be confused as to whether or not I'm in my house that I grew up in, or in a home like I'm in now. I have to really concentrate to remember the phones. Sometimes I'll forget where the phone is.

Derealization Severity Rating—Severe. Ms. S.'s derealization is rated as severe because her symptoms are recurrent. In addition, the *nature* of her derealization (she is confused about the reality of her immediate surroundings) also qualifies her symptom as severe. (See Severity Rating Definitions for further information.)

4. Identity confusion. Ms. S.'s answers during this section of the interview indicate that she has persistent confusion regarding her identity. In response to Question 101, she describes recurrent feelings of internal discord and fierce conflict:

Interviewer: Have you ever felt as if there was a struggle going on inside of you?
Patient: Yeah.
Interviewer: What's that like?
Patient: A war, it's a war.
Interviewer: Can you describe that some more?
Patient: It's as if I have several levels of consciousness and they all have an equal amount of, um *[pauses]* what it takes to be, an equal amount of what it takes to be a human being, bear a name. They argue and they pull and struggle and battle.
Interviewer: And when you say "they," what are you referring to?
Patient: The different levels of consciousness. It's levels, that's how I think of it.
Interviewer: How often do you have that feeling?
Patient: A lot.

This excerpt illustrates the interviewer's flexibility in inviting Ms. S. to elaborate further on her experiences of identity confusion. Because dissociative symptoms are often slippery or hard to describe, patients may develop their own images or metaphors for the different parts or aspects of themselves. Ms. S. experiences her internal loss of coherence as a struggle between "different levels of consciousness." The interviewer gives her the opportunity to clarify the meaning of that expression for herself. Patients often remark during feedback interviews that one of the most helpful and educative aspects of the SCID-D for them is the chance to define or "name" their dissociative experiences.

Ms. S. mentions further that her episodes of identity confusion affect her functioning to the point of immobilizing her in the most literal sense:

Interviewer: Are there any physical symptoms that accompany that struggle inside of you?

Patient: Yeah. It's like not being able to breathe, and the anxiety. I find myself crawling on the floor. I find myself in the corner.

Interviewer: So you find yourself crawling on the floor when you're home?

Patient: Yeah.

Interviewer: And you feel that it might be related to the struggle?

Patient: I feel—I know.

Interviewer: You *know* that it is related to the struggle.

Patient: Yeah.

Interviewer: Have you ever felt confused as to who you are?

Patient: *[pauses]* Yeah.

Interviewer: What is that like?

Patient: Um, I have to remind myself that I'm 36 and not back at home as a child.

Interviewer: Adolescents and other individuals may have periods of identity confusion. How does your confusion compare with that experience by others that you know?

Patient: Um, my feelings—it's with me all the time and it immobilizes me.

Interviewer: So, literally the feeling immobilizes you? Or symbolically?

Patient: No, literally. Yeah.

Again, Ms. S.'s description suggests the presence of age regression and identity alteration, as well as identity confusion.

Identity confusion Severity Rating—Severe. Due to the persistent and recurrent nature of Ms. S.'s identity confusion, this symptom is rated as severe. (See Severity Rating Definitions for further information.)

5. Identity alteration. Ms. S. reports several external behavioral manifestations of identity alteration. Some of these are evident to others, who have commented on them to her. She reports that "most people" who know her have remarked that she acts like a different person from time to time.

At an earlier point in the interview, Ms. S. indicated that she has been puzzled for some time by episodes of uncharacteristic behavior that have hurt others and that felt alien to her:

Patient: I said something that I didn't mean and that was very offensive, that hurt someone, and *I* wouldn't have said it. It's just very uncharacteristic for me to have done that.

Interviewer: How often would you say that experience occurs?

Patient: That I did that? I think it probably happens a lot more than I know now, now that I look back on things that have happened.

In addition, Ms. S. endorses other symptoms of identity alteration. In reply to Question 122, she reports that she has found items in her possession, such as furniture, lamps, clothes, and shoes, that she cannot recall having purchased. Moreover, she indicates in response to Question 135 that she has noticed alterations in her learned skills:

Interviewer: Have you ever experienced rapid changes in your capabilities or ability to function?

Patient: When I was younger, tests, I would take tests and I didn't know where the answers were coming from, but they would come. And then at other times I wouldn't be able to do it at all.

Interviewer: It would be the same course all the time?

Patient: Oh no.

Interviewer: Different courses?

Patient: Yeah. I would get an A in Spanish and then

I would get the exam, and I wouldn't be able to tell you how I got that A. The same thing in meetings, the different things that I go to now [in the course of my job]. Sometimes in these meetings, I will end up realizing that I participated a whole lot and had a whole lot of valuable input, but if you were to ask me to do it, I couldn't do it.

Interviewer: Do you mean you couldn't do it? Or do you mean that you couldn't recall what valuable input you had?

Patient: I couldn't remember doing it and I couldn't do it.

This excerpt is an instructive example of the interconnection of dissociative symptoms: Ms. S. is providing the interviewer with evidence that there are amnestic barriers between some of her internal parts. Additionally, she acknowledges that she refers to herself by several different names (Alice, Bobby, Susan, and Michelle), that others have called her by some of these names, and that she associates these names with distinctive behaviors, including self-injury. Ms. S. is also supplying confirmation that her references to "going inside" during earlier sections of the SCID-D are connected to episodes of identity alteration:

Interviewer: Does Alice or Bobbie or Susan or Elaine ever take control of your behavior or your speech?

Patient: Oh yeah.

Interviewer: What's that like? How does that occur?

Patient: Um, I don't know how it occurs, but I go inside. Um, Elaine will have sex. Elaine eats. Elaine grocery shops. Elaine has friends at the music school. Elaine has had a relationship, a friendship, relationship with some piano teacher at the music school. Um, things like that.

Interviewer: So when Elaine is in control you're more . . .

Patient: Alice went to school, you know, went to college.

Interviewer: Michelle?

Patient: Michelle burned me.

Interviewer: What did she burn you with?

Patient: A cigarette lighter and lighted cigarettes.

Identity alteration Severity Rating—Severe. The use of several different names to refer to oneself is listed in the severity rating definitions as one manifestation of severe identity alteration. Furthermore, Ms. S. said she did this several times per week. In addition, the fluctuations in Ms. S.'s level of functioning and specific skills, together with finding unexplained clothing and furniture in her possession, qualify her identity alteration as severe. (See Severity Rating Definitions for further information.)

Summary of Dissociative Symptoms

Ms. S. has each of the five dissociative symptoms at a high level of severity. She has large gaps in her memory, reports weekly depersonalization, frequent derealization, daily episodes of identity confusion, and a significant degree of identity alteration, including the use of several names. In addition, she also experiences ongoing dialogues between herself and the other personalities.

Interviewer: When you say that you have dialogues, is it a back-and-forth type of dialogue?

Patient: Yeah. Mmhmm. One part will say, "How could you do that?" and the other part will answer. The other part will say, you know, whatever the answer.

Interviewer: Are the dialogues similar to thoughts, or is there an auditory component to it that's similar to hearing a voice?

Patient: Oh, oh, I hear them. I hear the voices; they have different sounds.

Interviewer: How do they sound differently?

Patient: Um, Susan sounds young, um, Elaine sounds older and more carefree. Bobbie sounds older than Susan, but yet there's still a child quality in her voice.

Summary of Information Obtained From the Follow-Up Section of the SCID-D

The interviewer administered the follow-up section on different names, because this seemed the most direct section for further elaboration of the extent of identity confusion and alteration.

Ms. S. mentions that "Susan" has short hair and "likes to suck her thumb and play in a tub." Elaine likes to "go out, shops, drinks, is outgoing." "Her tone of voice is different and she has long hair." Susan is associated with a younger age and "talks like a 7-year-old," whereas Bobbie is "up to age 12." Ms. S. has ongoing dialogues between these people and reports that they have spoken directly to her therapist. She believes that they have different feelings and states emphatically that "they are separate." During the follow-up section, the interviewer observed changes in Ms. S.'s demeanor, speech, and physical posture consistent with her description of her child alter "Susan." These behaviors included curling up in a chair and sucking her thumb.

In summary, we learn that this patient has ongoing dialogues with these different personalities. The names are associated with consistent visual images, ages, behaviors, and feelings that are different from the patient's. In addition, Ms. S. reports that they have spoken with her therapist. She was also observed to change her behavior to that of a young child. Thus, the interviewer is given further indication of severe identity alteration.

Diagnostic Assessment and Differential Diagnosis

1. Does the patient appear to have a Dissociative Disorder, past or present? This patient suffers from all five dissociative symptoms, in the severe form. In the follow-up section, we learn that she also experiences severe identity fragmentation, the existence of different people within her. She believes they have different memories and they feel separate rather than a part of her identity. Ms. S. does appear to have a Dissociative Disorder according to DSM-IV criteria.

2. Which of the Dissociative Disorders should be in the differential diagnoses? The DSM-IV criteria for the five Dissociative Disorders are included here to help you follow the interviewer's process of differential diagnosis:

DSM-IV Diagnostic Criteria for Dissociative Amnesia

A. The predominant disturbance is one or more episodes of inability to recall important personal information, usually of a traumatic or stressful nature, that is too extensive to be explained by ordinary forgetfulness.

B. The disturbance does not occur exclusively during the course of Dissociative Identity Disorder, Dissociative Fugue, Posttraumatic Stress Disorder, Acute Stress Disorder, or Somatization Disorder and is not due to the direct physiological effects of a substance (e.g., a drug of abuse, a medication) or a neurological or other general medical condition (e.g., Amnestic Disorder Due to Head Trauma).

C. The symptoms cause clinically significant distress or impairment in social, occupational, or other important areas of functioning.

Ms. S. has had numerous experiences that meet Criterion A for Dissociative Amnesia, such as forgetting items of basic personal information, as well as episodes of time loss in the course of doing household chores. However, her amnesia cannot be regarded as the predominant symptom, because it occurs in conjunction with other dissociative symptoms, such as depersonalization and identity alteration. Thus, she does not meet Criterion A.

DSM-IV Diagnostic Criteria for Dissociative Fugue

A. The predominant disturbance is sudden, unexpected travel away from home or one's customary place of work, with inability to recall one's past.

B. Confusion about personal identity or assumption of a new identity (partial or complete).

C. The disturbance does not occur exclusively during the course of Dissociative Identity Disorder and is not due to the direct physiological effects of a substance (e.g., a drug of abuse, a medication) or a general medical condition (e.g., temporal lobe epilepsy).

D. The symptoms cause clinically significant distress or impairment in social, occupational, or other important areas of functioning.

Dissociative fugue involves the interaction of three SCID-D symptoms: amnesia, identity confusion, and identity alteration.

Although Ms. S. did report that she sometimes "found [her]self" in her therapist's office or shopping without remembering how she got there, she also answered "no" to subsequent questions related to fugue (Questions 9 and 11); therefore, follow-up fugue questions were not explored. She subsequently fails to meet Criteria A and B of Dissociative Fugue (and Criteria C and D are now irrelevant).

DSM-IV Diagnostic Criteria for Depersonalization Disorder

A. Persistent or recurrent experiences of feeling detached from, and as if one is an outside observer of, one's mental processes or body (e.g., feeling like one is in a dream).

B. During the depersonalization experience, reality testing remains intact.

C. The depersonalization causes clinically significant distress or impairment in social, occupational, or other important areas of functioning.

D. The depersonalization experience does not occur exclusively during the course of another mental disorder, such as Schizophrenia, Panic Disorder, Acute Stress Disorder, or another Dissociative Disorder, and is not due to the direct physiological effects of a substance (e.g., a drug of abuse, a medication) or a general medical condition (e.g., temporal lobe epilepsy).

Ms. S. meets Criteria A, B, and C for Depersonalization Disorder. She describes episodes of "going through the motions" and feeling like a detached observer of her own life. She also reports a high level of distress caused by her depersonalization. Furthermore, although these experiences are upsetting to her, they do not involve evidence of psychosis. On the other hand, Ms. S. cannot be said to meet Criterion D. Although she does not have depersonalization secondary to a substance use disorder or a medical problem, her symptoms do fit the criteria for Dissociative Identity Disorder.

Syndrome With Derealization (Dissociative Disorder Not Otherwise Specified)

When evaluating the symptom of derealization, the diagnosis of Dissociative Disorder Not Otherwise Specified (DDNOS) should be included in the differential diagnosis. DSM-IV includes derealization unaccompanied by depersonalization within the description of DDNOS, explained more fully as "disorders in which the predominant feature is a dissociative symptom . . . that does not meet the criteria for any specific Dissociative Disorder" (p. 490).

Although Ms. S. has severe derealization, she has also endorsed persistent and equally severe depersonalization. Thus, the "derealization without depersonalization" subcategory of DDNOS does not apply. In addition, the interviewer has obtained sufficient information from the administration of the optional follow-up sections to ascertain that Ms. S. also has severe identity alteration. Her alternate personalities are sufficiently distinct to assume different names, ages, and personality traits, such that she perceives them as "separate." Thus, Ms. S. does not fit the subcategory of DDNOS described as "presentations in which a) there are not two or more distinct personality states, or b) amnesia for important personal information does not occur."

DSM-IV Diagnostic Criteria for Dissociative Identity Disorder (Multiple Personality Disorder)

A. The presence of two or more distinct identities or personality states (each with its own relatively enduring pattern of perceiving, relating to, and thinking about the environment and self).

B. At least two of these identities or personality states recurrently take control of the person's behavior.

C. Inability to recall important personal information that is too extensive to be explained by ordinary forgetfulness.

D. The disturbance is not due to the direct physiological effects of a substance (e.g., blackouts or chaotic behavior during Alcohol Intoxication) or a general medical condition (e.g., complex partial seizures). **Note:** In children, the symptoms are not attributable to imaginary playmates or other fantasy play.

Ms. S. answered the SCID-D items such that all of these criteria were satisfied. Based on this interview, this patient meets the criteria for Dissociative Identity Disorder. The diagnosis of Dissociative Identity Disorder clearly subsumes the DDNOS disorders involving cases similar to Dissociative Identity Disorder but lacking some defining features. And more inclusively, Dissociative Identity Disorder, being the most severe dissociative syndrome, subsumes any and all of the other Dissociative Disorders.

3. Is there any reason why a Dissociative Disorder should be excluded in this patient? No. There is no evidence of a psychotic disorder such as schizophrenia, and Ms. S.'s reality testing appears intact. Also, the patient denies use of drugs and alcohol or any history of acute medical illness.

4. The Summary Score Sheet. Finally we have all the information necessary to complete the Summary Score Sheet, which is found on the last page of the interview (see completed sample in Appendix 1). It is useful to fill out this summary sheet while referring back to items in each symptom area. A rating of severe for each dissociative symptom is checked off, and finally "presence of Dissociative Disorder" and "Dissociative Identity Disorder" is checked off. This sheet is a compact synopsis of the patient's interview results and diagnosis. At a glance, the severities of the five symptoms and, if applicable, the type of Dissociative Disorder can be seen.

Case 2: The Angry Genie in the Bottle

Case 2, "The Angry Genie in the Bottle," concerns a patient with a history of temper outbursts and alcohol abuse, whose underlying Dissociative Disorder had never been previously identified.

Sample SCID-D Psychological Report for Inclusion in Patient Records

Summary of Evaluation: Paul L.

Dates of evaluation. 4/7/92, 4/14/92.

Referral source. Self-referred.

Chief complaint. Mr. L. presented to the walk-in clinic at General Hospital requesting outpatient treatment for "temper outbursts that I can't control." The patient complained that these outbursts, which usually occur at work, are followed by equally intense bouts of depression. He also complained of difficulty falling asleep at night.

History of present illness. Mr. L. is a 30-year-old, unmarried auto mechanic of French-Canadian background working in Holyoke, Massachusetts, and living with his parents in Granby, Massachusetts. He reports that his "temper outbursts" have occurred several times a year since adolescence. However, due to an increase in their frequency during the past month to weekly occurrences, the temper tantrums are now causing friction with his parents and employer. These episodes include inappropriately angry reactions to benign comments or questions from co-workers, screaming at himself for trivial mistakes or spillages, and swearing at customers. Mr. L. also has periods of "lost time" at work, lasting for an hour or two, three or four times a week, that are not related to substance abuse or seizures. He has no history of head injury other than childhood beatings of unclear frequency, nor any record of military service.

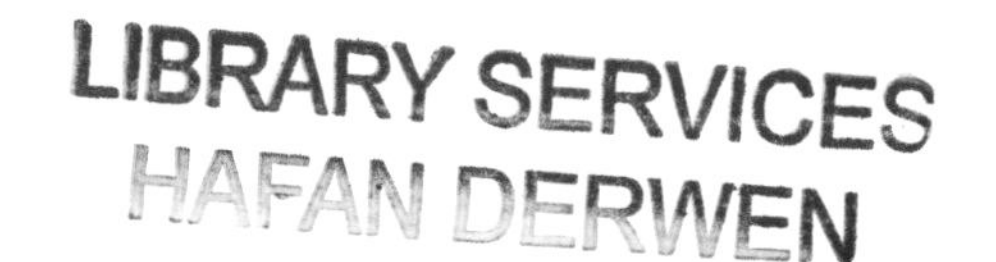

Psychiatric history. Mr. L. reports a history of intermittent alcohol abuse since adolescence. He was hospitalized twice for treatment of alcohol abuse (in 1984 and 1989) in an alcohol inpatient unit in Northampton. He was hospitalized for a month each time. He denies ever having used other drugs. He also has a history of three brief outpatient therapies, each lasting for approximately 6 months, for treatment of his present complaints. He reports that in the past, he has been treated with Mellaril, 25 mg prn, for relief of his agitation. At present, Mr. L. has been abstinent from alcohol for 2 years.

Family history. Mr. L., who is the third son in a family of six children, endorsed a history of verbal and physical abuse at the hands of several family members, going back to his early childhood. His father is an alcoholic who has never received treatment. Paul spoke of his immediate family as a "house divided" and a "hostile environment." He described in detail one episode when he was in junior high in which a next-door neighbor slammed him repeatedly against a brick wall for cutting across his backyard; Mr. L.'s older brother had urged the neighbor to "finish him off." Mr. L. describes his mother as verbally critical and recounts instances of her calling him a "hoodlum" or questioning his sanity. The patient also remarked that he felt "rejected and hurt" as a child by his family and that his present temper outbursts are triggered by feelings of rejection. In addition to family, Mr. L. also felt picked on or rejected by classmates in school for a mild speech impediment and minor dental malocclusion. He believes that his present shyness with women is due to these longstanding feelings of social inadequacy. His parents, now retired, continue to ridicule and criticize him for his mood swings and "crazy" behavior. His father is still actively drinking and frequently invites the patient to drink to keep him company.

Mental status examination. Mr. L. was casually dressed in a short-sleeved shirt and jeans, maintained good eye contact, and was cooperative throughout the interview. His speech was fluent, and there was no evidence of psychosis. His mood fluctuated between depression and overt anger. He gave relevant answers to the interview questions and was without looseness of associations or tangential thinking. Mr. L. denied visual hallucinations or hearing voices, with the exception of hearing his name called occasionally at work and assuming his co-workers were calling him. He endorsed having the Schneiderian symptoms of thought insertion and thought withdrawal. He reported chronic feelings of intermittent depression and feelings of worthlessness. He denied suicidal ideation but did acknowledge intense angry feelings related to fear that "Angry Paul" might take control of his behavior and hurt someone.

SCID-D evaluation summary. In addition to performing a routine diagnostic evaluation, I administered the *Structured Clinical Interview for DSM-IV Dissociative Disorders* (SCID-D) (Steinberg 1994b) to systematically evaluate posttraumatic dissociative symptoms and the presence of a Dissociative Disorder. The SCID-D was then scored according to the guidelines described in the *Interviewer's Guide to the SCID-D* (Steinberg 1994a). A review of the significant findings from the SCID-D interview includes the following:

> Mr. L. has chronic amnestic episodes that last for several hours, three to four times a week, that involve his forgetting his age as well as his actions, behaviors, and appointments with others during the lost time. The patient also endorsed experiences of depersonalization that include feelings of detachment from his behavior and feelings that his body is foreign to him.
>
> During this section of the interview, he expressed feelings of a split between a participating and observing self in terms of "an angry man with burning green eyes, like lasers," inside him, who tries to force him to "let [him] out" or who engages in a wrestling contest with Paul. He reported that his depersonalization episodes occurred several times per week, and prior to the

last 2 years, he would drink alcohol in an attempt to alleviate these feelings.

With respect to the symptom of derealization, Mr. L. described frequent experiences of feeling that his surroundings were unreal. With regard to symptoms of identity disturbance, the patient mentioned having had an imaginary companion in childhood, who remained with him through his adolescent years. Mr. L. also endorsed the use of different names for himself, including the first names of famous movie stars and baseball players. He occasionally has dialogues with himself using these names.

During the follow-up sections of the interview, Mr. L. described "Angry Paul" as a separate character. He repeatedly expressed fears that Angry Paul would "get outside" and take control of his behavior, including doing serious injury to others. Mr. L. mentioned that Angry Paul is triggered by experiences of social rejection or criticism. The patient denied that the other names are separate personalities; he considers them "parts of [him]self."

Assessment. Based on the SCID-D evaluation, Mr. L.'s symptoms are consistent with a primary diagnosis of a Dissociative Disorder. The predominant feature of his disturbance includes recurrent episodes of amnesia, depersonalization, derealization, and identity confusion, each rated as severe on the SCID-D. More specifically, his symptoms meet DSM-IV criteria for Dissociative Disorder Not Otherwise Specified, which cover cases that are similar to Dissociative Identity Disorder but that fail to meet full criteria for this disorder. Examples include cases in which "there are not two or more distinct personality states," or "amnesia for important personal information does not occur" (DSM-IV, p. 490).

It is not clear on the basis of this interview whether Angry Paul is a distinct alter personality or a personality fragment representing one aspect of Mr. L.'s emotions. However, the results of the SCID-D indicate that the patient's disruptive temper outbursts are most likely manifestations of Angry Paul. Mr. L.'s alcohol abuse appears to be secondary to a primary Dissociative Disorder.

Recommendation. I recommend the following: 1) outpatient therapy with a clinician knowledgeable about the treatment of dissociative symptoms and disorders; 2) initial treatment focus on patient education, including the nature of the dissociative symptoms and identification of their triggers; 3) reviewing techniques for behavioral control of the dissociative symptoms, as well as improved cooperation with Angry Paul; 4) a follow-up administration of the SCID-D in 6 months to monitor symptoms and rule out Dissociative Identity Disorder (a subset of patients with Dissociative Identity Disorder may present first with symptoms consistent with Dissociative Disorder Not Otherwise Specified); and 5) use of an antianxiety agent as needed for symptomatic relief of anxiety associated with dissociative symptoms.

Case 3: The Man Without a Past

Unlike the patient in Case 2, the patient in Case 3 had no history of outpatient or inpatient therapy prior to the onset of massive amnesia following an episode of fainting. His is an illustrative example of the SCID-D's ability to detect the presence of a Dissociative Disorder in a patient who presents with symptoms suggestive of a medical illness.

Sample SCID-D Psychological Report for Inclusion in Patient Records

Summary of Evaluation: Frank R.

Dates of evaluation. 10/10/92; 10/17/92.

Referral sources. Linda Jensen, M.D. (psychiatrist); Brian McDonald, M.D. (neurologist).

Reason for referral. Diagnostic evaluation; neurologist suspects presence of dissociative disturbance.

Information obtained from: Frank, current psychiatrist, neurological report, and patient's wife.

Brief summary. Frank R. is a 41-year-old owner of a small business in Chicago, Illinois, who resides with his wife and three children in Lake Forest, Illinois. Mr. R. was referred for psychiatric diagnostic evaluation following an episode of syncope that occurred in his home on 8/2/92, followed by global retrograde amnesia. Immediately following his fainting episode, he was taken to a local emergency room where he received a comprehensive medical evaluation. Physical and neurological examination were unremarkable, and all laboratory tests and a computed tomography scan were within normal limits. He was referred for an EEG with nasopharyngeal leads that was subsequently performed on an outpatient basis; this also was without abnormal findings. The patient has no history of substance abuse, is not a military veteran, and has no known medical problems other than an allergy to ragweed pollen.

The patient has no history of psychiatric disturbance and is currently in outpatient treatment with Dr. Jensen for the amnesia. He is distressed about his inability to recover his memory, particularly because there are no apparent immediate stressors severe enough to account for either the fainting or the amnesia. He also acknowledged recent attacks of agoraphobia, including fear of driving further than 5 miles from his house. His wife accompanied him to the interview because of his fear of driving. She cannot recall any events in her husband's life that could be considered traumatic, although she did mention that he was a professional athlete for about 10 years before he changed careers and opened his present business. She is co-owner of the business and indicates that it has succeeded to the point of adding three new employees in the past year.

Psychiatric history. Mr. R.'s only hospitalization was following his "fainting" episode and subsequent global amnesia. He was hospitalized for 4 weeks (8/2/92–8/31/92) and treated with psychotherapy, without medication. His discharge diagnosis was Psychogenic Amnesia. On discharge, he was referred to Dr. Jensen for outpatient treatment.

Family history. Due to his global amnesia, Mr. R. was unable to provide information regarding his childhood or parents, stating that he could not remember the details of his childhood relationships. He was able to report that he is the oldest of six children and that he felt he had been punished by physical beatings by his father at unclear intervals of frequency. He completed 3 years of college and has been married to his present wife since 1973. They have three daughters, ages 18, 15, and 11 years. He reports that the marriage has been stable, with no separations. The oldest daughter is in college in Michigan, and the younger two reside at home. He indicated that his wife and all three children have been supportive throughout his hospitalization and his present inability to work.

Mental status examination. Mr. R. was neatly dressed in casual clothing. He was calm and cooperative, although his anxiety level increased noticeably toward the end of the interview as it began to get dark outside. He spoke clearly and intelligently and answered the interviewer's questions with relevant replies. His overall mood appeared euthymic. He reported hearing voices associated with inner dialogues and denied suicidal or homicidal ideation. Mr. R. also reported feeling depressed about his recent inability to function but denied vegetative symptoms. For a complete summary of Mr. R.'s dissociative symptoms, see the evaluation below.

Evaluation summary. In addition to performing a routine mental status examination, I administered the *Structured Clinical Interview for DSM-IV Dissociative Disorders* (SCID-D) (Steinberg 1994b) to systematically evaluate the patient's dissociative symptoms and the presence of Dissociative Disorders. The SCID-D was then scored according to the guidelines described in the *Interviewer's Guide to the SCID-D* (Steinberg 1994a). A review of the significant findings from the SCID-D interview includes the following:

> Mr. R. has severe retrograde amnesia that affects his recall of almost all of his life prior to 8/2/92, with the exception of information supplied by his wife and other family members and a few memories of major events such as his wedding. There is no evidence of anterograde amnesia. He experiences recurrent episodes of depersonalization, which include seeing himself sitting in two different chairs simultaneously and feeling divided between participating in life and being an observer of it from the outside.
>
> With regard to the symptom of derealization, the patient endorsed frequent episodes of feeling that his surroundings seemed unreal. He associated this feeling with episodes of "trances," which sometimes lasted for 1–2 hours. Although Mr. R. denied having panic attacks, he did state that the trances cause him severe anxiety, which keeps him from working and going about his usual activities. With respect to identity confusion, Mr. R. reported that he experienced an ongoing struggle between a side of him that wanted to regain his memory and a side that did not want to have memories of his past. He reported experiencing dialogues between these two sides in which he would find himself arguing with himself about whether or not today would be the day he would regain his memory for his entire past. With regard to the symptom of identity alteration, Mr. R. endorsed feeling as if he was acting like a different person since his memory loss, in that he was not able to function as he had previously. In addition, he endorsed experiencing episodes during which he would feel like he was a child and find himself crawling around his home.
>
> During the SCID-D follow-up section, Frank reported seeing and talking to "dark beings" in his trance states who resemble humans, although they do not have distinctive faces or clothing. He maintains that these beings can talk to his wife and therapist and that they have told the therapist that they are stronger than he is. Mr. R. also described feeling "frightened of the dark" and was reassured that his wife was waiting for him and would drive him home.

Assessment. Based on this evaluation, Mr. R.'s symptoms since his hospitalization are consistent with a primary diagnosis of a Dissociative Disorder. More specifically, his experiences of severe amnesia, depersonalization, derealization, identity confusion, and identity alteration, as well as recurrent trance states, are consistent with a diagnosis of Dissociative Disorder Not Otherwise Specified (DDNOS). Mr. R.'s symptoms fit the subcategory of DDNOS specified by DSM-IV, which covers cases similar to Dissociative Identity Disorder but that fail to meet full criteria for this disorder. Examples include cases in which "there are not two or more distinct personality states," or "amnesia for important personal information does not occur" (DSM-IV, p. 490). His global amnesia has resulted in regressed childlike behavior involving dependence on his wife or elderly parents and fears of the dark. His regressed functioning in turn has caused feelings of depression and anxiety.

Recommendation. I recommend individual therapy focused on treatment of the full range of Mr. R.'s dissociative symptoms. Initial treatment goals would include 1) patient education regarding these symptoms, and review of specific techniques for alleviating them (i.e., grounding techniques to alleviate his depersonalization and derealization episodes); and 2) exploration of the inner dialogues and dark beings, insofar as fostering cooperation among these inner voices may assist Mr. R. in recovering memories of his past. It appears that the emergence of a childlike part in Mr. R., which currently controls his behavior, is related to a struggle between functioning as a responsible adult (with memories of his adult existence) and functioning as a child, with behaviors and fears associated with his childhood (and no memories of his adult existence).

Second, Mr. R. should receive a follow-up administration of the SCID-D in 6 months to monitor his symptoms and to rule out Dissociative Identity Disorder, insofar as a subset of patients with Dissociative Identity Disorder may present initially with symptoms consistent with DDNOS. Mr. R.'s anxiety and depression appear to be secondary to his dissociative symptoms. The use of an antianxiety agent as needed may assist in alleviating his anxiety.

Case 4: The Postman Rings Twice

Carol N. was referred for diagnostic consultation by her therapist, who suspected the presence of dissociative symptoms. Ms. S.'s responses to the SCID-D are used to illustrate and review the use of the instrument in differential diagnosis and assessment, from the assessment of the severity of her dissociative symptoms to the final diagnosis.

Demographic History, History of Present Illness, and Psychiatric History

Carol N. is a 25-year-old, single, white woman who lives with her parents in a remote area of California. She was diagnosed in infancy as having petit mal seizures but was referred for diagnostic evaluation by her therapist and neurologist because of symptoms that were atypical of epilepsy. According to the patient, her seizures remitted when she was 18 months old and returned when she was age 12. At the time of the interview, she described her symptoms as "uncontrolled"; she reported that her "seizures" now consisted of experiences of "jolting awake," with "body shaking," about four nights a week. The patient expanded on these experiences as including feelings of "being suffocated," "feeling like I'm having a heart attack," "feeling paralyzed," and "screaming 'No!'." In addition to her seizure symptoms, Ms. N. also had one experience of head injury in childhood, when she tumbled from a bed in the course of roughhousing with her siblings. She required stitches for the cut in her scalp but denied loss of consciousness. Last, Ms. N. mentioned episodes of self-injury; when asked to describe what she meant by "trying to harm herself," she specified drinking liquid soap, attempting to jump out of a moving car, and running in front of cars.

Ms. N. presented as a pleasant but subdued young woman, fashionably attired with a shawl, jewelry, and dark nail polish complementing her dress. She occasionally twisted the ends of the shawl during the interview. Her voice was soft, high-pitched, and slightly childlike. Although her general speech patterns and vocabulary were those of a well-read and articulate person, her self-descriptions throughout the interview indicated a persistent underestimation of her intelligence and talents. She indicated that she had dropped out of college after her second year.

Ms. N. first presented for psychiatric treatment at age 24, when she was hospitalized for 3 weeks due to depression and suicidal ideation. Her first frightening encounter with her dissociative symptoms occurred after her discharge from the hospital, when she walked to a shopping plaza from her parents' house, wrote checks recorded in her checkbook for items that she could not recall purchasing, and wandered the area for some time unable to remember her name, address, or telephone number. Personnel from the hospital where she had been committed were able to identify her. At the time of the SCID-D interview, Ms. N. had been in outpatient therapy with a psychiatric social worker for 10 months.

Medications

Ms. N. was taking the following medications daily at the time of the interview: Tegretol (anticonvulsant), 400 mg/day; Prozac (antidepressant), 20 mg; and Ativan (anxiolytic), 0.5 mg. She had been treated with phenobarbital to control her seizures at the time she was first diagnosed with epilepsy; the medication was discontinued several years later after her seizures stopped.

Family History

Ms. N. endorsed a history of alcohol abuse in both parents, which began when they were separated for a year because of the father's employment. She was 8 years old when he was sent to Europe for a year by his corporation. The patient remarked that her father has been drunk numerous times in the presence of other family members. She also indicated that her mother had a history of depression, and that her father is "maybe a little paranoid." Neither parent has ever been treated for their psychiatric symptoms or for their substance abuse.

During the SCID-D interview, Ms. N. spontaneously supplied some details of her family's verbal abuse of her, such as her parents' calling her "airhead" and "stupid," and other derogatory comments about her intelligence and maturity. She endorsed a history of verbal abuse by her parents as constant since childhood; she added that they abused her siblings in this way as well. The patient used the metaphor of a "minefield" to define the emotional atmosphere of her household. Ms. N. expanded on her family's negative reactions to her illness, commenting that they tell her repeatedly that she is "a pain to live with." She also reported having been sexually abused, although she was unsure of her age at the time of the assault(s) or of the perpetrator's identity. In addition, a pattern of revictimization is present in her history; she indicated that she was raped by a former landlord and two of his "friends" when she was 22.

The material that follows includes a review of Ms. N.'s dissociative symptoms as assessed with the SCID-D, severity ratings of her symptoms and the considerations relevant to differential diagnosis, including substance use, organic disorders, and psychotic disorders.

Assessment of the Five Dissociative Symptoms

1. Amnesia. In response to Question 1 ("Have you ever felt as if there were large gaps in your memory?"), Ms. N. reports experiencing significant memory deficits. She found herself "not remembering weekends, weeks, months, years—people ask questions and you don't remember being with them, don't remember childhood occurrences that everybody else seems to remember." When asked about her educational history, she indicated that she had no recollection of large blocks of her schooling, from junior high school through college. She could not remember how many times this has occurred: "I really can't determine time." She reported that her time gaps were "really scary" and that she would call a crisis hotline when "coming to" (i.e., regaining "consciousness"), not being able to remember what she had been doing for the last several hours. On one occasion, she "came to" in a local shopping mall, realized that she had missed an appointment with her therapist, and called him in a state of considerable anxiety.

Ms. N. also reported frequent episodes of finding herself in a place and not knowing how or why she went there (Question 7). She found herself in "San Diego, 'coming to' in a barbershop getting my hair cut. Why or how, I don't know." She said this type of experience occurred "at least a few times a week." When asked if she had ever found herself away from home, not knowing who she was (Question 11), she reported that she has experienced this often. She described being found wandering around town not knowing who she was and remembered often needing to look at her ID to determine her name, age, or address. She could not remember how many times this has happened. When asked if she has ever been unable to remember this basic personal information (Question 15), she said that it occurred "many times . . . every week." The patient mentioned that she compensates for her memory gaps by pretending that she recognizes people who claim to know her. In the follow-up section later in the interview, she remarked, "I don't really have memories. I can basically tell you what people have told me, and then I have a memory of that, but it's not the actual memory."

Ms. N. reports abstention from drugs or alcohol, so these amnestic episodes have occurred without the use of drugs or alcohol and in the absence of acute medical illness. She was consistent in her answers on both occasions when the interviewer asked her about her substance use. In addition, the patient's symptoms occur independently of her epilepsy and, in fact, were present even when she was seizure free.

Amnesia Severity Rating—Severe. Ms. N.'s amnesia is rated as severe because of its nature (not remembering weekends, weeks, months, years, not knowing who she was); frequency (weekly to daily gaps in her memory); and degree of accompanying distress ("really scary").

2. Depersonalization. Ms. N. endorsed numerous manifestations of depersonalization. She reported feeling as if she were watching herself from a point outside of her body (Question 38): "It's like sitting on my shoulder or like standing back, watching the scene." This occurred daily. When asked for how long she could remember this happening, she replied, "I don't know—ages." She answered whether she felt as if she were a stranger to herself (Question 40), in the affirmative: "It's a little weird, feeling that your body doesn't belong to you—someone else's face, someone else's face in the mirror, someone else's voice, someone else's thoughts. It's frustrating. You feel trapped." Ms. N. also endorsed the feeling that part of her body is foreign (Question 41): "The hands look strange, or the arms look strange . . . The touch—it didn't feel like *I* was touching me. It was someone else that was touching me. The perceptions were different. It just didn't seem right."

She mentioned feeling that her whole being was unreal (Question 44). It was "scary, depressing, very depressing. . . . It felt like just going through the motions, like the whole world was foreign or I was foreign to the whole world. It was just different." Last, Ms. N. answered that she felt that she was going through the motions of living but that the real self was far away (Question 46). She experienced this as "watching us having a conversation with somebody . . . like watching a movie . . . like you're on the movie screen or something. It's hard to explain." She mentioned that this occurred weekly.

The patient's answers to this section of the SCID-D are of interest to clinicians because they exemplify the ways in which the instrument's open-ended format encourages patients to provide additional relevant information. For instance, Ms. N. complained of a headache during this part of the assessment interview and added that she usually experiences such headaches "right before things become strange—you know, tunnel vision, increased hearing, and things like that." She appears to be describing perceptual distortions that occur in conjunction with a derealization episode. Second, the patient begins to describe the impact of dissociative symptomatology: she has found her symptoms "puzzling, very puzzling," but it has taken her years to realize that "everybody doesn't feel this way. I thought it was just one of the quirks of life." Note that this attitude of resignation and helplessness is one reason why so many people with Dissociative Disorders have been diagnosed with depression. In addition, Ms. N.'s comments exemplify the fact that many patients with Dissociative Disorders become habituated to their symptoms to the extent that they no longer feel disquieted by them. Ms. N. stated that she was "not really uncomfortable [with a feeling of depersonalization] because I've felt it so often. I'm only uncomfortable now that I realize it's not normal." Third, she also remarked in more detail about the effects of her disorder on her relationships and consequent negative feedback from significant others. She reported not only that episodes of depersonalization interfere with her relationships because she has to "work hard at concentrating" when they occur, but also that she has "heavy mood swings, radical mood swings that people complain about." The patient's episodes of depersonalization have occurred without the use of drugs or alcohol and in the absence of acute medical illness. Again, she consistently reports never using drugs or alcohol, and her symptoms are not related to her epilepsy.

Depersonalization Severity Rating—Severe. Ms. N.'s depersonalization is rated as severe due to a variety of factors, including its frequent recurrence (weekly), the degree of distress caused ("scary, depressing"), and the extent of dysfunctionality (difficulty concentrating).

3. Derealization. On the third section of the assessment interview, Ms. N. endorsed derealization episodes in which familiar surroundings and people felt unreal or unfamiliar (Question 79). She stated, "My room seems unreal, unfamiliar, my closet, my family . . . mother father, brother, sister . . . they seem unfamiliar." These experiences occurred on a weekly basis. When asked if anyone in particular seemed unreal to her, she replied, "My father."

Ms. N. also described being unable to recognize close friends, relatives, and her own home (Question 82). She recounted "walking down the street toward a group of friends and not recognizing them until they stop and . . . start talking to me and then I realize that, oh, maybe I know these people." In other instances, she remembers: "I don't drive—my friends drive me places—going home, saying they haven't been to my house before, and I can't find it. You stall and drive around for a little while until you remember which one it is, or you say, 'Oh, I have to do a chore,' and do something else, you know, without telling them." Episodes like these occur monthly. In addition, Ms. N. reported feeling puzzled as to what is real and unreal in her surroundings (Question 84): "It's like I'm in a dream sometimes. Knowing that it's real but it doesn't seem unreal." She could not recall how often that particular form of derealization occurs.

Again, it is significant that the patient expressed harsh self-judgments during this section of the interview. When asked by the interviewer, "How do you understand that feeling [of not recognizing family members]?," Ms. N. replied, "I don't [understand it]. I just thought I was an airhead—some strange psychotic person or something." Derealization enables individuals to distance themselves from their family, as can be gauged from her remark that "a lot of times it seems like I'm not a part of the family." She indicated that she felt that way at least once a week.

Derealization Severity Rating—Severe. This symptom is rated as severe because her derealization is recurrent and results in significant social dysfunction, as measured, for example, by her reluctance to drive. In addition, the *nature* of her derealization (she has been unable to recognize her father, close friends, and her home) is also severe.

4. Identity confusion. The fourth section of the SCID-D interview indicates that Ms. N. has persistent confusion regarding her identity. When asked if a struggle was going on inside of her (Question 101), she replied: "Yes . . . a struggle for identity, who I am, what I'm like, attitudes, beliefs, knowledge . . . not knowing who I am—identity—you know, our name is Carol, but it doesn't seem like our name. Does that make sense? We're trying to figure out what that is." This struggle occurs almost daily. She experienced these feelings as "threatening, scary, and very frustrating. Sort of like being in a candy store and not being able to decide which candy."

Ms. N. also responded that she felt confused as to who she really was (Question 102). Her descriptions included experiences of sexual identity confusion: "Not knowing even what it's like to be a woman. Not even really knowing. I know I have all the body parts, but what is that? Not knowing what I truly feel, not being able to decide on—just—a lot. . . . Well, I know, on forms, we checked 'Female,' because we have, you know, those parts, but not knowing really what it's like to be a female? Not even really the slightest idea." The difficulty patients often have in expressing symptoms of identity confusion is exemplified by her comment: "I'm totally puzzled—neutral. I can't even describe it. I just don't know. I just don't know. I don't." Note that sexual identity confusion and a general numbing of sexual feelings are common sequelae of childhood sexual abuse, which the patient endorsed.

Identity confusion Severity Rating—Severe. Due to the persistent nature of her identity confusion, as well as its associated distress, this symptom is rated as severe. The nature of the identity confusion (regarding all aspects of her identity, including sexual) also yields a rating of severe.

5. Identity alteration. Ms. N. endorses several significant subjective and behavioral manifestations of identity alteration. When asked if she ever felt as if or found herself acting as if she were still a child (Question 113), she responded, "Yes," and described it as "very puzzling. Very confusing. You know, realizing that you shouldn't go around carrying a teddy bear." She reported that others criticized her childlike views and behaviors: "People saying to 'Grow up! Why are you behaving like this?'—things like that." She also remembers "coming to" in a toy store playing with toys, "things like that." She reported that episodes of this nature occur weekly.

When the interviewer asked her if she ever acted as if she were a completely different person (Question 114), she responded: "Yeah . . . coming to in a bar, talking to a bunch of guys, that I had no idea who they are. Things like that. And then withdrawing, you know, going back, again, where you're watching. And that's the last memory." That occurs "every once in a while, that I'm, you know, aware of." In addition, she reported being told by others that she seemed like a different person (Question 116): "Yes . . . a friend of mine, Doug, he'll often say, 'Who are you? I don't know this Carol. Who are you?'"—particularly when she does not remember experiences they had together that were important to him. She experienced his reactions as "distressing" and "scary." She then mentioned that "family, friends remark on mood changes that had happened that day, 'Why are you doing that? I don't understand you. Who are you?' type of thing." Ms. N. also mentioned her boyfriend's incomprehension mixed with anger when she could not recall their sexual activity during one of their dates. Although her comment was in reply to a question about identity alteration, it clearly reflects her amnesia as well.

Ms. N. endorsed having referred to herself by different names (Question 118), but only through confirmation from others: "Recently we've—we [laughs]—have been told that [we] refer [to ourselves] in the plural sense once in a while, and Carol is a common one at work that the girls hear. But I don't remember doing it." The patient reported that co-workers and fellow students had occasionally called her by different names (Question 120): "They've called me Jamie, Vinnie, Carol, Anne, Gloria, things like that." Additionally, "Carol and Vinnie receive mail." She could remember being called these names since grade school. Her family also called her those names. When the interviewer asked if she knew the people who sent mail to the other names, she replied, "Sometimes I do, sometimes I don't. There are still a few letters that I haven't figured out who's what." She replied that when she gets the mail, "I take it upstairs to my room. Sometimes I read it and try to figure out what it is. I believe I wrote back a couple of times trying to figure out who was what, but I keep getting mail, so, I don't know . . . I would say it's an even third of the mail." She added that mail addressed to her other names has been coming to her house over a period of years.

Ms. N. also recalled finding things in her possession that seemed to belong to her but that she could not remember purchasing (Question 122): "There are a lot of different toiletries. Several different perfumes. You know, lingerie that I would never imagine getting. Clothes, dresses, that I would never consider buying . . . all different styles. Young, old, tacky, tacky as in cheap." This occurs "a lot," although she believes she's not conscious of many of her shopping expeditions.

She also described another personality who did not have a given name: "There's one I refer to as the Screamer, which is totally screaming. Can't stop it . . . [I] get mad at somebody and blow up more than you should, but watching myself yell at this person and realizing that this isn't the way it should be. Scaring friends when that happens. They don't know who I am. You know, they jump back."

Identity alteration Severity Rating—Severe. The use of several different names to refer to oneself is listed in the SCID-D's Severity Rating Definitions as a manifestation of severe identity alteration. Receiving mail addressed to these names is another indication of severe identity alteration. Other endorsements indicating severe identity alteration in conjunction with amnesia include recurrent episodes of acting like a different person and finding unfamiliar items in her room.

Associated Features of Identity Disturbance

Mood changes. Ms. N. mentioned having rapid mood changes at several points during the assessment interview but gave the most detailed answer to Question 134. She reported that her moods fluctuated "from very calm and peaceful to very violent, angry, to crying, temper tantrums, like a little kid." When asked how often these mood changes occurred, she responded, "I would say daily."

Internal dialogues. The patient also reported the presence of ongoing internal dialogues (Question 138). She remarked that these dialogues "help me with information. Just talk. How to do things, what to do, little squabbles with myself. I've never really thought about it." These dialogues occurred daily. When asked at this point if she was having an internal dialogue during the interview itself, she replied, "Off and on." Responses of this type should be noted in the scoring of a patient's intra-interview dissociative cues after the interview has been concluded. These endorsements, including frequent mood fluctuation and age regression, are further indications of identity confusion and alteration.

Summary of Dissociative Symptoms

Ms. N. has each of the five dissociative symptoms at a severe level. She has large gaps in her memory and reports weekly episodes of depersonalization and derealization, daily episodes of identity confusion, and a marked degree of identity alteration. Her endorsement of identity alteration includes the use of several names, accompanied by daily internal dialogues, a feeling of being controlled, and daily rapid mood changes. The existence of all five dissociative symptoms at a high level of severity is typical of Dissociative Identity Disorder or Dissociative Disorder Not Otherwise Specified (DDNOS), both of which require additional information on identity confusion and identity alteration. The necessary supplemental material can be obtained by administration of the appropriate follow-up sections.

Follow-Up Sections on Identity Confusion and Identity Alteration

The interviewer first administered the follow-up section on "Different Names" (Questions 192–201) because it seemed to be the most direct follow-up section for further elaboration of the extent of identity confusion and alteration, based on the patient's previous responses. The interviewer said, "Earlier you did mention that others have referred to you by different names: Vinnie and Jamie and Carol and Gloria. Can you say some more about these names?" (elaboration on Question 192). She replied, "I go along whenever a stranger calls me by these names. Trying to figure out what's going on."

When Ms. N. was asked whether she felt as if "the names" she mentioned ever controlled the way she acted or talked (Question 193), she answered, "Yeah . . . being out of control of your voice, and things like that—your thoughts. Racing to get a thought out, but someone else gets the voice first." When asked how her voice changed, she replied, "Whiny, up and down, you know, deep low." When the interviewer inquired as to whether she had visual images of the names (Question 194), she replied, "Different variations. Sometimes of me, sometimes of I don't know who. This is really touchy. I can't say." The patient then mentioned that she was having internal dialogues at this point, which were interfering with her responses to the interviewer. Ms. N. added that there were different ages associated with the names (Question 195): "I'd say it's 4 to 8 to 13 to 15, different stages . . . Anne [is age 4] . . . Jamie would be 8 to 13. *[pause]* Now it's getting all muddled . . . I can't grasp it. It's really weird. Sometimes thoughts come in and then they go away. It's like I'm not supposed to know or something." She mentioned earlier in the interview that she pictured one of her child parts as "scared, lonely, and hurt," and that Anne was "scared." The interviewer then asked, "If Anne could speak, what would be said?" (Question 197). Ms. N. replied, "Anne would cry." She also mentioned that Vinnie and Jamie could talk to her therapist directly (Question 198). She then described Jamie as "athletic . . . and he likes wood."

The patient was then asked whether the memories, behaviors, or feelings of the names were different from her own, and she replied, "Different." She mentioned that the voices inside made her aware of that, as well as the letters she received that were addressed to the different names and were written in different styles: "Vinnie is a more spiritual, asexual type, and Carol seems to be more flirtatious." She felt that the names were separate as opposed to part of her personality (Question 200). At this point, the interviewer concluded the interview, having decided that a second set of follow-up questions was unnecessary; the patient had already provided responses indicating severe levels of identity confusion and alteration.

In summary, we learn that Ms. N. associates "the names" (or the personalities) with consistent behaviors, memories, and feelings that are different from her own. She reports that some of the identities have spoken with her therapist and that they seem separate from her personality. The interview has now ended, and the interviewer rates one section before making a diagnosis.

Intra-Interview Dissociative Cues

After the conclusion of the interview, the interviewer rated the patient for intra-interview dissociative cues—that is, behaviors and symptoms observed during the interview that are suggestive of dissociative symptomatology and/or disorder. Thirteen items are listed in this section of the SCID-D. The interviewer takes both verbal statements and the patient's visual appearance into account in completing this section. In this particular assessment, the interviewer did notice an alteration in the subject's demeanor and mood (Items 259–262). Ms. N. was also observed to refer to herself in the first-person plural (Item 263). Additionally, she often omitted pronouns altogether when talking about herself, suggesting confusion regarding self-reference. The patient also reported intra-interview internal dialogues (Item 264). Ms. N. exhibited intra-interview amnesia (Item 265), particularly when answering chronicity questions. She gave many responses like "I do not know" or "I do not remember" to basic questions (Item 268). In addition, the patient gave ambivalent responses to questions about dissociative symptoms (Item 269) as seen in her pausing, her comments that "someone" was telling her not to answer, and her occasional "uh-oh's," as if she were unsure of the safety of being honest during the interview. Moreover, Ms. N. responded with a significant degree of emotion to questions regarding dissociative symptoms (Item 270), as indicated by her sad mood, lengthy pauses, and occasional sighs. No hypnotic eye movements were observed (Item 271); however, she did have a slight trancelike or glassy-eyed appearance (Item 272).

Differential Diagnosis

Ms. N. had been referred by her therapist and neurologist for a consultation to rule out the presence of a Dissociative Disorder. During the assessment and feedback interviews, her diagnosis was reviewed, and a course of treatment was recommended. Because accurate diagnosis is the primary step toward effective treatment of Dissociative Disorders, an outline of the interviewer's process of differential diagnosis follows.

Dissociative Amnesia. The presence of severe amnesia warrants consideration of the possible diagnosis of Dissociative Amnesia. DSM-IV criteria for Dissociative Amnesia are

A. The predominant disturbance is one or more episodes of inability to recall important personal information, usually of a traumatic or stressful nature, that is too extensive to be explained by ordinary forgetfulness.

B. The disturbance does not occur exclusively during the course of Dissociative Identity Disorder, Dissociative Fugue, Posttraumatic Stress Disorder, Acute Stress Disorder, or Somatization Disorder and is not due to the direct physiological effects of a substance (e.g., a drug of abuse, a medication) or a neurological or other general medical condition (e.g., Amnestic Disorder Due to Head Trauma).

C. The symptoms cause clinically significant distress or impairment in social, occupational, or other important areas of functioning.

This patient has had numerous episodes that appear to meet Criterion A for Dissociative Amnesia, such as losing years of time and being unable to remember her age or address. However, her amnesia symptoms are not isolated occurrences, because they occur in conjunction with the other four dissociative symptoms. Thus, Dissociative Amnesia cannot be viewed as her predominant disturbance.

Dissociative Fugue. Dissociative Fugue involves the interaction of three symptoms assessed by the SCID-D—amnesia, identity confusion, and identity alteration. The criteria for Dissociative Fugue as specified by DSM-IV are

A. The predominant disturbance is sudden, unexpected travel away from home or one's customary place of work, with inability to recall one's past.

B. Confusion about personal identity or assumption of a new identity (partial or complete).

C. The disturbance does not occur exclusively during the course of Dissociative Identity Disorder and is not due to the direct physiological effects of a substance (e.g., a drug of abuse, a medication) or a general medical condition (e.g., temporal lobe epilepsy).

D. The symptoms cause clinically significant distress or impairment in social, occupational, or other important areas of functioning.

The patient endorsed Question 11 (traveling away from home and forgetting who she was) in support of Criteria A and B. However, the fugue episodes in this patient are not isolated events; they occur in the context of the other dissociative symptoms assessed by the SCID-D. As a result, fugue cannot be described as this patient's predominant disturbance, and therefore she does not meet Criterion A for Dissociative Fugue.

Depersonalization Disorder. The DSM-IV criteria for Depersonalization Disorder are

A. Persistent or recurrent experiences of feeling detached from, and as if one is an outside observer of, one's mental processes or body (e.g., feeling like one is in a dream).

B. During the depersonalization experience, reality testing remains intact.

C. The depersonalization causes clinically significant distress or impairment in social, occupational, or other important areas of functioning.

D. The depersonalization experience does not occur exclusively during the course of another mental disorder, such as Schizophrenia, Panic Disorder, Acute Stress Disorder, or another Dissociative Disorder, and is not due to the direct physiological effects of a substance (e.g., a drug of abuse, a medication) or a general medical condition (e.g., temporal lobe epilepsy).

Criterion A is satisfied by Ms. N.'s recurrent episodes of depersonalization, including feelings of unreality, foreignness, and being an external observer. Her reality testing was intact during these episodes, thus meeting Criterion B, as indicated by her lucidity and lack of delusions during her experiences of depersonalization. Marked distress and social impairment were evident in her descriptions, satisfying Criterion C. Criterion D is not met because she meets the criteria for Dissociative Identity Disorder (see below).

Derealization Without Depersonalization: Dissociative Disorder Not Otherwise Specified. When evaluating the symptom of derealization, the interviewer should include the possibility of Dissociative Disorder Not Otherwise Specified (DDNOS) in the differential diagnosis. DSM-IV lists "derealization unaccompanied by depersonalization in adults" as Example 2 under the heading of DDNOS, which is described more fully as "disorders in which the predominant feature is a dissociative symptom (i.e., a disruption in the usually integrative functions of consciousness, memory, identity, or perception of the environment) that does not meet the criteria for a specific dissociative disorder" (DSM-IV, p. 490).

Although this patient has derealization, she also has persistent episodes of severe depersonalization. Therefore, the classification "derealization unaccompanied by depersonalization in adults" is not applicable, and DDNOS can be excluded from the differential diagnosis.

Dissociative Identity Disorder (Multiple Personality Disorder). When a patient experiences a moderate-to-severe level of identity confusion, the interviewer should include Dissociative Identity Disorder and DDNOS in the differential diagnosis. To explore this symptom and these syndromes further, refer to the SCID-D's "Identity Alteration" section, the associated features of identity disturbance, and follow-up sections on identity confusion and alteration. The diagnosis of Dissociative Identity Disorder subsumes the diagnosis of DDNOS, as well as the other three Dissociative Disorders.

The criteria for Dissociative Identity Disorder as specified by DSM-IV are

A. The presence of two or more distinct identities or personality states (each with its own relatively enduring pattern of perceiving, relating to, and thinking about the environment and self).

B. At least two of these identities or personality states recurrently take control of the person's behavior.

C. Inability to recall important personal information that is too extensive to be explained by ordinary forgetfulness.

D. The disturbance is not due to the direct physiological effects of a substance (e.g., blackouts or chaotic behavior during Alcohol Intoxication) or a general medical condition (e.g., complex partial seizures). **Note:** In children, the symptoms are not attributable to imaginary playmates or other fantasy play.

It is obvious from Ms. N.'s answers to a number of questions in the SCID-D interview that she meets Criteria A and B for Dissociative Identity Disorder. She has mentioned the existence of alternate personalities with distinct names, ages, character traits, and genders; in addition, she receives mail addressed to some of these alters and has found items in her possession that were acquired when another personality was in control of her behavior. Additional evidence that she meets Criterion B has been supplied by friends and family members, in the form of comments that she acts like a different person with them from time to time. Criterion C is met by her episodes of severe amnesia, such as her "coming to" in cities several hundred miles away from her home and needing to check her own ID to remind herself of her name, age, and home address. Ms. N.'s abstinence from alcohol and drugs, together with the fact that her dissociative symptoms occur independently of her epilepsy, satisfies Criterion D. In sum, Ms. N.'s symptoms are consistent with a diagnosis of Dissociative Identity Disorder, which subsumes the diagnoses of other Dissociative Disorders.

Clinical Applications of the SCID-D and Treatment Planning

In addition to differential diagnosis, the SCID-D is useful to clinicians in screening for specific symptoms because it allows them to monitor the patient's progress with regard to them. It is then possible to set specific treatment goals for diminishing the severity of each of the five dissociative symptoms.

Patient Education

Educating patients about the nature and prognosis of their symptoms is an important dimension of any treatment plan for recovery from a Dissociative Disorder. Precisely because these disorders are distinctive among psychiatric disturbances in that they have good prognoses in most cases, clinicians should be careful to inform patients of their diagnosis. This is particularly important when the patient has a lengthy history of trauma. Because of the social consequences of dissociative symptomatology (i.e., patients' frequent difficulties with employment and intimate relationships), accurate information concerning the nature and severity of the symptoms is necessary for improvement on the interpersonal as well as the intrapsychic level. Ms. N.'s case is particularly instructive in its reflection of the contribution of negative reactions from family and friends to the patient's general attitude of depression and personal inadequacy. Consequently, it is also a useful example of the critical position of patient education in the recovery process.

The feedback interview that followed administration of the SCID-D is an illustration of a patient's first tentative steps toward empowerment and self-affirmation. At first skeptical of the interviewer's estimation of her as "bright," Ms. N. proceeds to take a number of conversational initiatives in the course of the interview, asking questions about the necessity of recovering painful memories and of allowing her alters to identify themselves to her therapist, about the significance of her episodes of self-cutting, about the possible presence of dissociative disturbances in other family members, and about ways and means of explaining her disorder to her family. That all these insights and inquiries have arisen in her mind within a week of the SCID-D's administration is an indication of the interview's effectiveness as an educational tool and a diagnostic instrument. Although her low self-esteem and underestimation of her intelligence cannot be expected to dissipate overnight, it is evident from her genuine curiosity and desire to understand herself better, together with her active engagement with the interviewer, that she is on the path to recovery of confidence in her mental capacities, as well as cognitive integration of them.

Sample SCID-D Evaluation Report for Inclusion in Patient Records

Summary of Evaluation: Carol N.

Dates of evaluation. 2/20/93, 2/27/93, with Carol.

Referral sources. Martin Stone, M.S.W.; Jane Doe, M.D. (neurologist).

Reason for referral. Diagnostic evaluation, suspects presence of dissociative symptoms that cannot be accounted for by patient's history of epilepsy.

Information obtained from: Carol, current therapist, and referring neurologist.

Brief summary. Carol N. is a 25-year-old, part-time secretary in Palm City, California, who resides with her parents in Los Santos, California. Ms. N. was referred for diagnostic evaluation because of dissociative symptoms that her neurologist felt were not due to her petit mal epilepsy. She has a history of self-destructive behaviors, including self-cutting and the swallowing of household cleaners. She is currently in treatment with Mr. Stone on a once-weekly basis. She has reported instances of "coming to" in other cities on the West Coast, such as Seattle and San Diego, as well as finding herself in shopping malls, bars, etc. These episodes are unrelated to substance abuse or epileptic seizures and have been occurring over a period of years.

Psychiatric history. The patient was hospitalized for 3 weeks at Grove Village Hospital in 1990, followed by individual therapy with Mr. Stone. See reports from Grove Village Hospital for further details. Mr. Stone reports that he thinks the patient's current diagnosis is Borderline Personality Disorder.

Family history. Ms. N. described being subjected to verbal and sexual abuse in childhood and referred to alcohol abuse on the part of both parents beginning when she was age 10. She mentioned that her parents were separated for a year at this time due to the requirements of the father's employment. Ms. N. is the youngest of three children and has an older sister and an older brother. During the second interview on 2/27, the patient reported that her mother and sister manifest a variety of dissociative and compulsive symptoms. She indicated at that time that her family is not supportive of her problems, not well disposed toward psychotherapy in general, and inclined to ridicule or criticize her frequently.

SCID-D evaluation summary. In addition to performing a routine diagnostic evaluation, I administered the *Structured Clinical Interview for DSM-IV Dissociative Disorders* (SCID-D) (Steinberg 1994b) to systematically evaluate posttraumatic dissociative symptoms and the presence of Dissociative Disorders. The SCID-D was then scored according to the guidelines described in the *Interviewer's Guide to the SCID-D* (Steinberg 1994a). A review of the significant findings from the SCID-D includes the following:

> Ms. N. has severe amnestic episodes that occur on a daily or weekly basis and that involve losses of significant periods, including unexplained journeys and unaccountable purchases. She also experiences recurrent episodes of depersonalization that include feeling that her body does not belong to her, that "someone else" touches her, and that she is like an observer sitting on her own shoulder.
>
> In addition, Ms. N. endorses severe recurrent derealization and identity confusion, particularly confusion regarding her sexual identity. She reports episodes of identity alteration that include childlike behavior, mood swings that are confusing to her boyfriend and other friends, referring to herself by different names (including Vinnie, Jamie, Carol, and Gloria), and receiving mail addressed to these names.
>
> She also endorsed feeling controlled by these entities and experiencing them as separate from herself. Ms. N. was able to describe several examples of their control of her behavior, including speaking to her therapist and instances of self-cutting.

Mental status examination. Ms. N. was casually dressed in a conservative dress. She was calm and cooperative. She spoke clearly and intelligently and answered questions with relevant replies. She denied having any psychotic symptoms. She acknowledged intermittent feelings of depression that did not last for more than 2 weeks at a time; she also had episodic feelings of anxiety and panic. She felt that her moods were not in her control. Ms. N. has also had intermittent suicidal ideation and a history of self-destructive behaviors, including self-cutting, for which she has been amnestic. She denied acute suicidal or homicidal ideation. See the SCID-D Evaluation Summary for a description of Ms. N.'s dissociative symptoms.

Assessment. Based on this evaluation, Ms. N.'s symptoms and history of trauma are consistent with a primary diagnosis of a Dissociative Disorder. More particularly, her experiences of severe amnesia, depersonalization, derealization, identity confusion, and identity alteration consisting of the presence of several different alters who exist within her and assume executive control of her behavior are consistent with a diagnosis of Dissociative Identity Disorder. She also has a coexisting seizure disorder.

Recommendation. I recommend intensive individual therapy focused on treatment of the dissociative symptoms; specifically, the course of treatment should include educating the patient about the nature of her symptoms and helping her to identify the specific stimuli that trigger her amnesia, depersonalization, derealization, and identity alteration. This should be done to reduce the frequency and severity of her symptoms. Furthermore, I recommend exploration of the conflicts among her alter personalities to facilitate cooperation among them and to reduce the patient's self-destructive and self-mutilating behavior.

APPENDIX 1

Sample SCID-D Summary Score Sheet and Differential Diagnosis Decision Trees

Subject's initials C. S.
Interviewer M. Steinberg

Date 12/30/92
Total SCID-D score 20

Summary Score Sheet for the SCID-D

A. OVERALL DIAGNOSTIC IMPRESSION	☐ No evidence of a Dissociative Disorder ☑ Meets criteria for a Dissociative Disorder ☑ Past episode ☑ Present ☐ Meets criteria for Acute Stress Disorder
B. TYPE OF DISSOCIATIVE DISORDER	☐ Dissociative Amnesia ☐ Dissociative Fugue ☑ Dissociative Identity Disorder (Multiple Personality Disorder) ☐ Depersonalization Disorder ☐ Dissociative Disorder Not Otherwise Specified

C. DISSOCIATIVE SYMPTOMS	Severity*	
AMNESIA	1 ☐ Absent 2 ☐ Mild 3 ☐ Moderate 4 ☑ Severe	☐ Only with alcohol or drugs ☐ Sometimes with alcohol or drugs ☑ Not associated with alcohol or drugs
DEPERSONALIZATION	1 ☐ Absent 2 ☐ Mild 3 ☐ Moderate 4 ☑ Severe	☐ Only with alcohol or drugs ☐ Sometimes with alcohol or drugs ☑ Not associated with alcohol or drugs
DEREALIZATION	1 ☐ Absent 2 ☐ Mild 3 ☐ Moderate 4 ☑ Severe	☐ Only with alcohol or drugs ☐ Sometimes with alcohol or drugs ☑ Not associated with alcohol or drugs
IDENTITY CONFUSION	1 ☐ Absent 2 ☐ Mild 3 ☐ Moderate 4 ☑ Severe	☐ Only with alcohol or drugs ☐ Sometimes with alcohol or drugs ☑ Not associated with alcohol or drugs
IDENTITY ALTERATION	1 ☐ Absent 2 ☐ Mild 3 ☐ Moderate 4 ☑ Severe	☐ Only with alcohol or drugs ☐ Sometimes with alcohol or drugs ☑ Not associated with alcohol or drugs

*See Severity Rating Definitions in the *Interviewer's Guide to the SCID-D*, Revised, pp. 18–22.

Scoring of the Summary Score Sheet for the SCID-D should be performed using the guidelines described in the *Interviewer's Guide to the Structured Clinical Interview for DSM-IV Dissociative Disorders* (SCID-D), Revised (Washington, DC, American Psychiatric Press, 1994. Copyright © 1985, 1993, 1994 Marlene Steinberg, M.D.).

FIGURE 4. SCID-D decision tree for the Dissociative Disorders. DID = Dissociative Identity Disorder. DDNOS = Dissociative Disorder Not Otherwise Specified.
Source. Reprinted with permission from Steinberg M: *Handbook for the Assessment of Dissociation: A Clinical Guide.* Washington, DC, American Psychiatric Press, 1995.

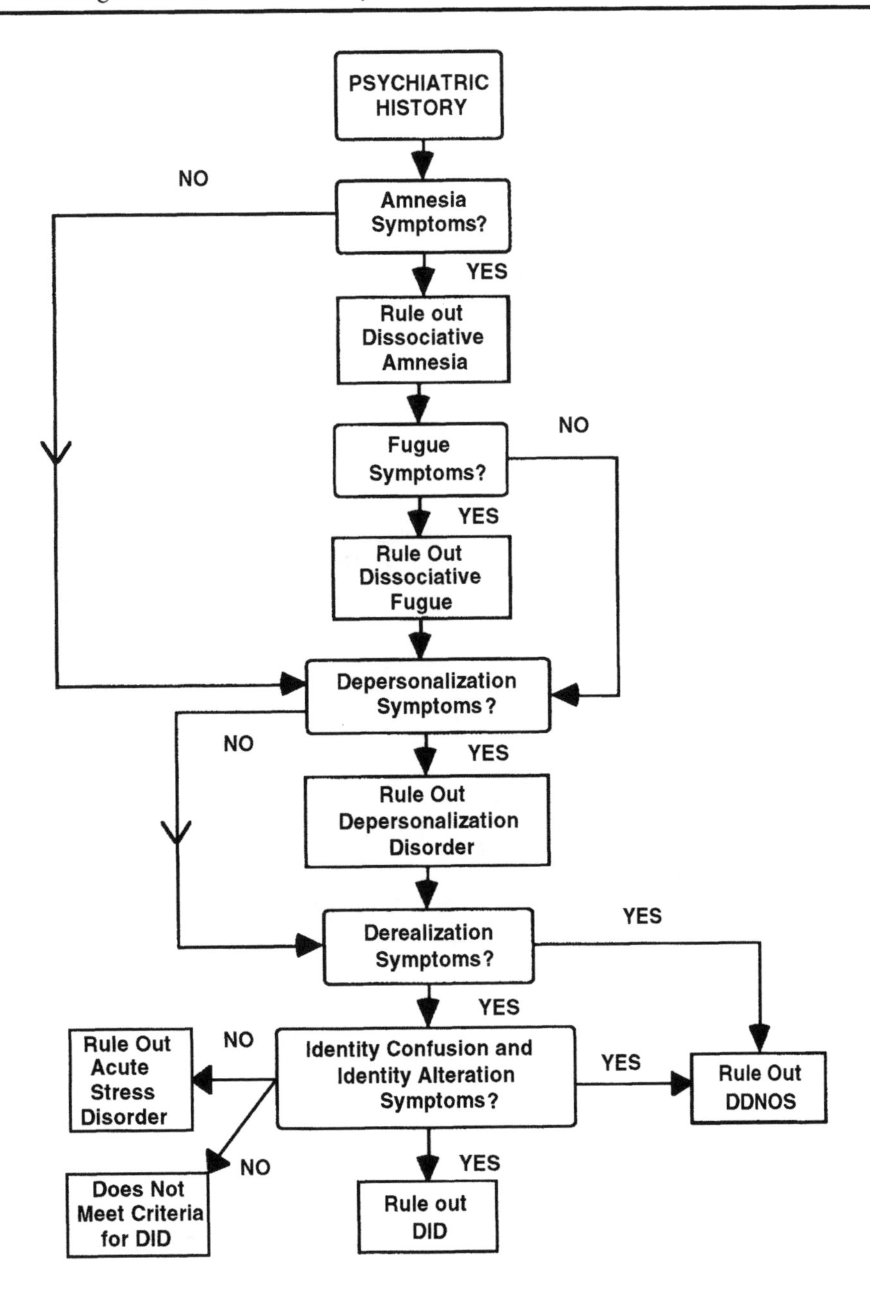

NOTE: The diagnosis of DID subsumes the diagnosis of any of the four Dissociative Disorders

FIGURE 5. SCID-D differential diagnosis decision tree for amnesia. DID = Dissociative Identity Disorder. DDNOS = Dissociative Disorder Not Otherwise Specified.

Source. Reprinted with permission from Steinberg M: *Handbook for the Assessment of Dissociation: A Clinical Guide.* Washington, DC, American Psychiatric Press, 1995.

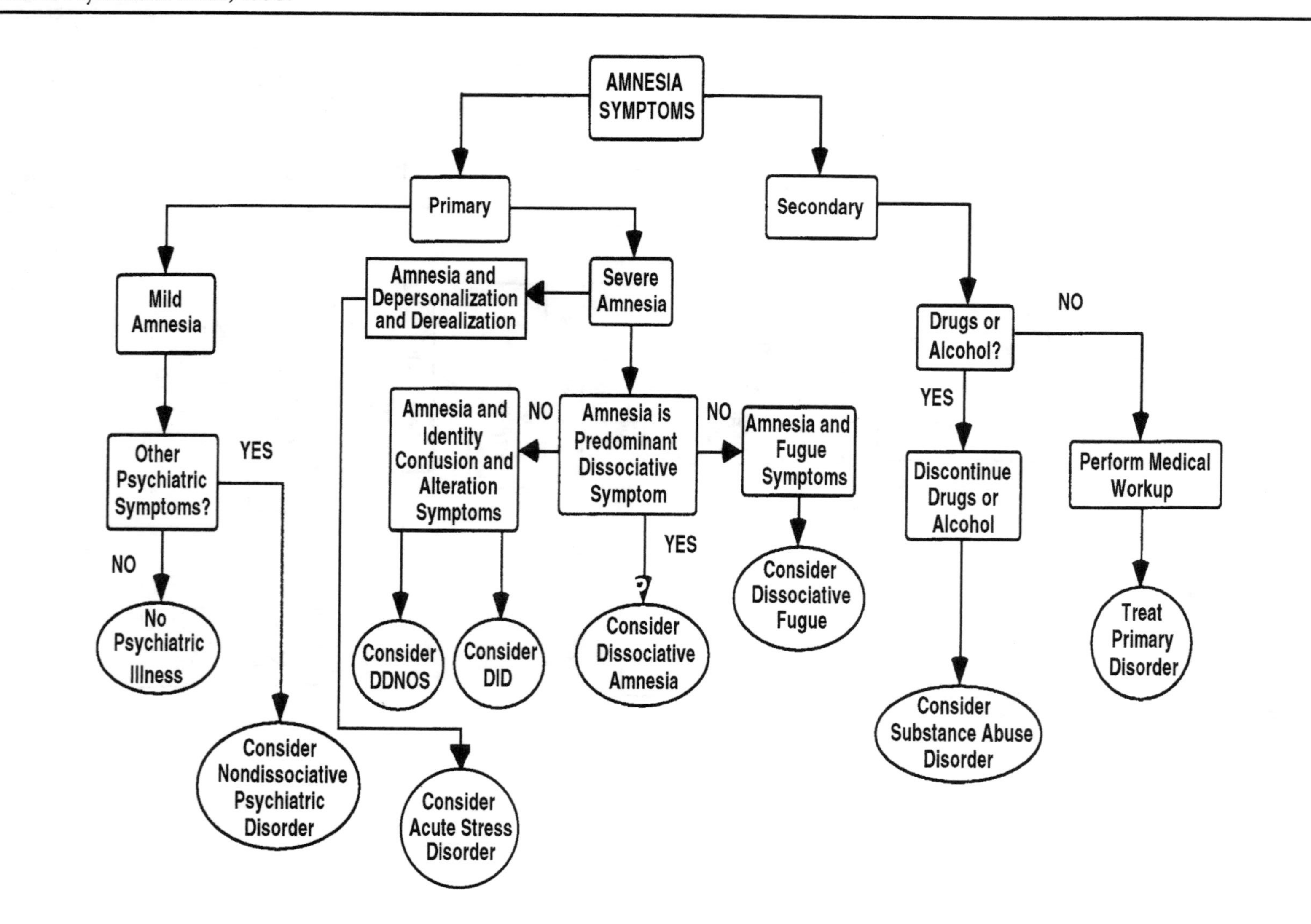

FIGURE 6. SCID-D differential diagnosis decision tree for dissociative symptoms. PTSD = Posttraumatic Stress Disorder.
Source. Reprinted with permission from Steinberg M: *Handbook for the Assessment of Dissociation: A Clinical Guide.* Washington, DC, American Psychiatric Press, 1995.

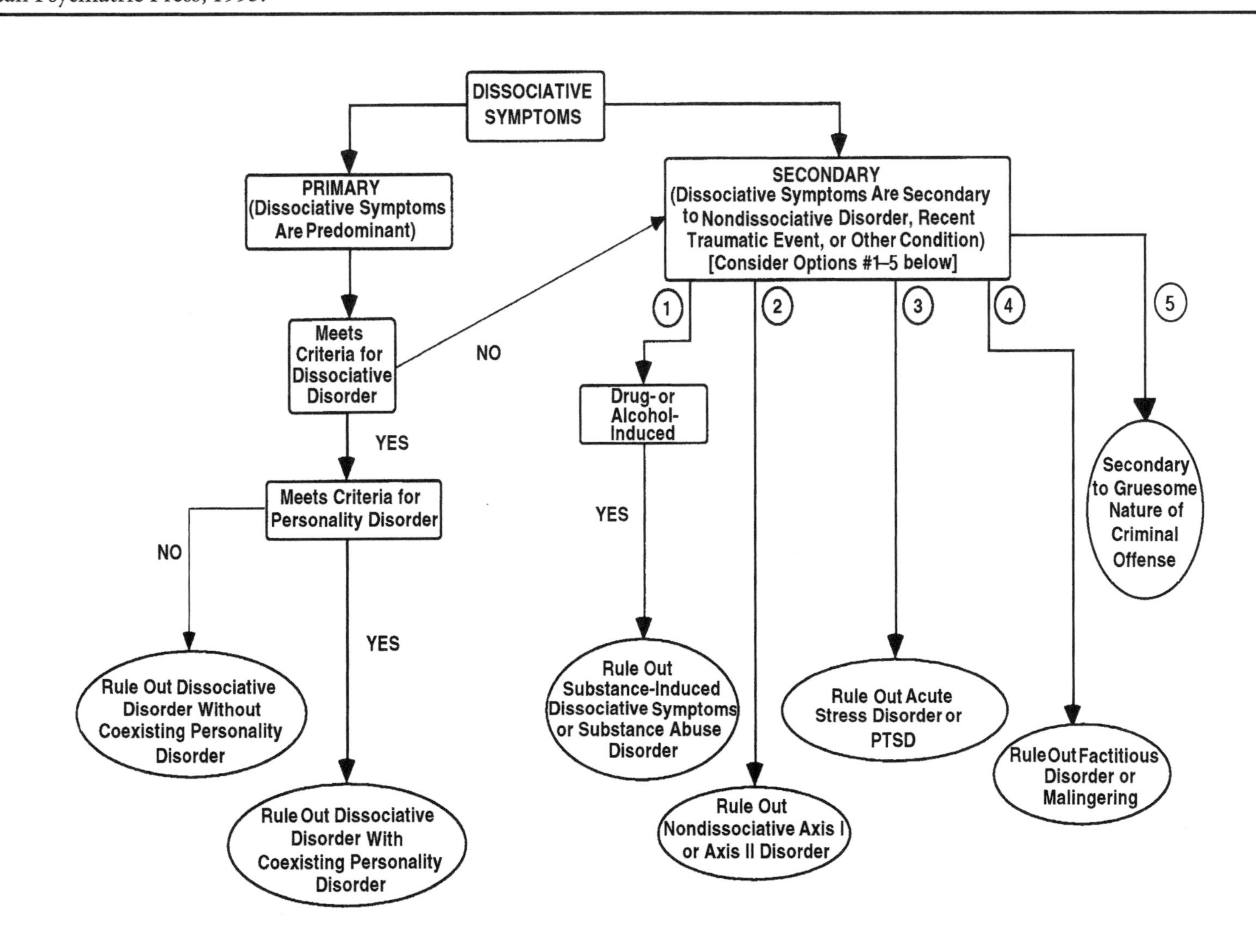

APPENDIX 2

Diagnostic Work Sheets

Subject's initials ______________ Date __________
Interviewer ______________

DISSOCIATIVE AMNESIA

Diagnostic Work Sheet

	SCID-D items	Yes	No
DSM-IV Criterion A for Dissociative Amnesia: A. The predominant disturbance is one or more episodes of inability to recall important personal information, usually of a traumatic or stressful nature, that is too extensive to be explained by ordinary forgetfulness.		____	____
SCID-D items supporting Criterion A: Both 1 and 2 must be present:			
1) Inability to recall important personal information. Amnesia is too extensive to be explained by ordinary forgetfulness; at least one of the following occurs:			
a) inability to recall one's identity	7, 15	____	____
b) inability to recall one's past (not associated with purposeful travel)	9	____	____
c) inability to recall other important personal information due to large memory gaps	1, 15	____	____
2) Memory loss was the predominant disturbance among all symptoms discussed and in the context of the subject's history.	1–17	____	____

DISSOCIATIVE AMNESIA
Diagnostic Work Sheet

	SCID-D items	Yes	No
DSM-IV Criterion B for Dissociative Amnesia:			
B. The disturbance does not occur exclusively during the course of Dissociative Identity Disorder, Dissociative Fugue, Posttraumatic Stress Disorder, Acute Stress Disorder, or Somatization Disorder and is not due to the direct physiological effects of a substance (e.g., a drug of abuse, a medication) or a neurological or other general medical condition (e.g., Amnestic Disorder Due to Head Trauma).		____	____
SCID-D items supporting Criterion B: All of the following must be present:			
1) The disturbance is not due to Dissociative Identity Disorder (confirm through ratings on Dissociative Identity Disorder Diagnostic Work Sheet).		____	____
2) The disturbance is not initiated and/or maintained exclusively by drugs, alcohol, serious head trauma, or medical illness.	24–28	____	____
DSM-IV Criterion C for Dissociative Amnesia:			
C. The symptoms cause clinically significant distress or impairment in social, occupational, or other important areas of functioning.			
SCID-D items supporting Criterion C:			
1) The amnesia causes marked distress or discomfort.	22–23	____	____
2) The amnesia interferes significantly with social relationships or ability to work.	21	____	____

DISSOCIATIVE AMNESIA
Diagnostic Work Sheet

	SCID-D items	Yes	No
SCID-D inclusion criteria based on severity and clinical significance of symptoms: The following constellation of clinically significant dissociative symptoms is present:			

	Symptom	Severity rating	Yes	No
i)	Amnesia	Severe	____	____
ii)	Depersonalization	Absent to Mild	____	____
iii)	Derealization	Absent to Mild	____	____
iv)	Identity confusion	Absent to Mild	____	____
v)	Identity alteration	Absent to Mild	____	____

(See SCID-D Severity Rating Definitions for further information.)

EXCLUSION CRITERIA FOR DISSOCIATIVE AMNESIA

Diagnostic Work Sheet

	SCID-D items	Yes	No
SCID-D exclusion criteria for Dissociative Amnesia: The presence of any of the following rules out the diagnosis of Dissociative Amnesia:			
A. Exclusion criteria regarding context and content of symptoms			
1) The following criteria, which suggest a diagnosis of organic mental syndrome or Dissociative Identity Disorder, exclude the diagnosis of Dissociative Amnesia:			
a) Amnesia was initiated exclusively by drugs, alcohol, serious head trauma, or medical illness.	24–28	____	____
b) Subject meets the criteria for Dissociative Identity Disorder or Dissociative Fugue. (See Dissociative Identity Disorder Diagnostic Work Sheet and Dissociative Fugue Diagnostic Work Sheet.)		____	____

Subject's initials ______________ Date ___________
Interviewer __________________

Dissociative Fugue

Diagnostic Work Sheet

	SCID-D items	Yes	No
DSM-IV Criterion A for Dissociative Fugue: A. The predominant disturbance is sudden, unexpected travel away from home or one's customary place of work, with inability to recall one's past.		____	____
SCID-D items supporting Criterion A: DSM-IV Criterion A, as indicated by the following:			
1) Unexpected travel away from home, with inability to recall one's past.	9, 11	____	____
2) Travel with memory loss for one's past is the predominant disturbance among all symptoms discussed in the interview and in the context of the patient's history.	9, 11 (all of interview)	____	____
DSM-IV Criterion B for Dissociative Fugue: B. Confusion about personal identity or assumption of new identity (partial or complete).		____	____
SCID-D items supporting Criterion B: DSM-IV Criterion B, as indicated by at least one of the following:			
1) Confusion about personal identity following sudden unexpected travel.	6, 7, 9, 11, 105	____	____
2) Assumption of a new identity (partial or complete) following sudden unexpected travel.	9, 11, 13	____	____

Dissociative Fugue
Diagnostic Work Sheet

	SCID-D items	Yes	No
DSM-IV Criterion C for Dissociative Fugue:			
C. The disturbance does not occur exclusively during the course of Dissociative Identity Disorder and is not due to the direct physiological effects of a substance (e.g., a drug of abuse, a medication) or a general medical condition (e.g., temporal lobe epilepsy).		____	____
SCID-D items supporting Criterion C: Both of these must be true:			
1) The disturbance is not due to Dissociative Identity Disorder. (See ratings on Dissociative Identity Disorder Diagnostic Work Sheet.)		____	____
2) The disturbance is not initiated and/or maintained exclusively by drugs, alcohol, serious head trauma, or medical illness.	31–35	____	____
DSM-IV Criterion D for Dissociative Fugue:			
D. The symptoms cause clinically significant distress or impairment in social, occupational, or other important areas of functioning.			
SCID-D items supporting Criterion D:			
1) The fugue symptoms cause marked distress or discomfort.	22,23	____	____
2) The fugue symptoms interfere significantly with social relationships or ability to work.	21	____	____

Dissociative Fugue

Diagnostic Work Sheet

	SCID-D items	Yes	No

SCID-D inclusion criteria based on severity and clinical significance of symptoms:
The following constellation of clinically significant dissociative symptoms is present:

	Symptom	Severity rating	Yes	No
i)	Amnesia*	Severe	____	____
ii)	Depersonalization	Absent to Mild	____	____
iii)	Derealization	Absent to Mild	____	____
iv)	Identity confusion Identity alteration*	Moderate to Severe in at least one of these symptoms	____	____

***Note:** In Dissociative Fugue, severe amnesia and identity alteration occur only in conjunction with the fugue.

(See SCID-D Severity Rating Definitions for further information.)

EXCLUSION CRITERIA FOR DISSOCIATIVE FUGUE

Diagnostic Work Sheet

	SCID-D items	Yes	No
SCID-D exclusion criteria for Dissociative Fugue: The presence of any of the following rules out the diagnosis of Dissociative Fugue:			
A. Exclusion criteria regarding context and content of symptoms			
1) The following criteria, which suggest a diagnosis of organic mental syndrome or Dissociative Identity Disorder, exclude the diagnosis of Dissociative Fugue:			
a) The predominant disturbance was initiated exclusively by drugs, alcohol, serious head trauma, medical illness, or seizure disorder.	31–35	____	____
b) Subject meets the criteria for Dissociative Identity Disorder. (See Dissociative Identity Disorder Diagnostic Work Sheet.)		____	____

Subject's initials ______________ Date ____________

Interviewer ________________

DISSOCIATIVE IDENTITY DISORDER

(MULTIPLE PERSONALITY DISORDER)

Diagnostic Work Sheet

	SCID-D items	Yes	No
DSM-IV Criterion A for Dissociative Identity Disorder:			
A. The presence of two or more distinct identities or personality states (each with its own relatively enduring pattern of perceiving, relating to, and thinking about the environment and self).		____	____
SCID-D items supporting Criterion A: The presence of at least three of the following four criteria indicates the presence of two or more distinct identities or personality states.			
1) Persistent feeling that two or more identities exist within him/herself, as indicated by at least one of the following:			
a) persistent feeling that he/she is two different people, one going through the motions of life and the other observing	46, 47	____	____
b) persistent feeling that he/she acts as if he/she were a different person or he/she is told by others that he/she seems like a different person	114, 116	____	____
c) use of different names, or being called by others by different names (not nicknames or an alias used only to facilitate illegal activity)	118, 120	____	____
2) Persistent manifestations of the presence of different personalities, as indicated by at least four of the following:			
a) ongoing dialogues between the different people	138–145 (see follow-up sections)	____	____
b) acting or feeling that the different people inside of him/her take control of his/her behavior or speech	(see follow-up sections)	____	____

Prepared for use in conjunction with Steinberg M: *Interviewer's Guide to the Structured Clinical Interview for DSM-IV Dissociative Disorders* (SCID-D), Revised. Washington, DC, American Psychiatric Press, 1994.

DISSOCIATIVE IDENTITY DISORDER

Diagnostic Work Sheet

	SCID-D items	Yes	No
c) characteristic visual image that is associated with the other person, distinct from subject	(see follow-up sections)	____	____
d) characteristic age associated with the different people inside of him/her	(see follow-up sections)	____	____
e) feeling that the different people inside of him/her have different memories, behaviors, and feelings	(see follow-up sections)	____	____
f) feeling that the different people inside of him/her are separate from his/her personality and have lives of their own	(see follow-up sections)	____	____
3) Associated features of Dissociative Identity Disorder as indicated by at least two of the following:			
a) recurrent amnestic episodes	1–7, 17	____	____
b) recurrent or persistent depersonalization	38–53	____	____
c) recurrent or persistent derealization	79–84	____	____
d) several depersonalization episodes that (one of the following):			
1. produce impairment in social or occupational functioning	63	____	____
2. are not precipitated by stressful events	64	____	____
3. are prolonged (lasting over 4 hours)	55, 56	____	____
e) rapid fluctuations in symptoms, mood, or level of functioning	134, 135	____	____
4) Intra-interview cues suggestive of Dissociative Disorder, as indicated by at least one of the following:			
a) marked alterations in subject's demeanor	259	____	____
b) alterations in subject's identity	260	____	____
c) spontaneous age regression	261	____	____
d) intra-interview amnesia	265	____	____
e) subject refers to him/herself in the third person	263	____	____
f) significant emotional response to SCID-D questions	270	____	____
g) trancelike appearance	272	____	____

Dissociative Identity Disorder

Diagnostic Work Sheet

	SCID-D items	Yes	No
DSM-IV Criterion B for Dissociative Identity Disorder: B. At least two of these identities or personality states recurrently take control of the person's behavior.		____	____
SCID-D items supporting Criterion B: The presence of at least one of the following supports DSM-IV Criterion B:			
1) History of alterations in his/her demeanor or identity, as if he/she were two different people.	113–116 (see follow-up sections)	____	____
2) Alterations in his/her speech (i.e., vocabulary, accents) and/or behavior that are not under his/her control.	(see follow-up sections)	____	____
3) Intra-interview manifestations of alterations in identity, as indicated by at least one of the following:			
a) dramatic alterations in subject's demeanor during interview	259	____	____
b) alterations in subject's identity	260	____	____
c) spontaneous age regression	261 (see follow-up sections)	____	____
DSM-IV Criterion C for Dissociative Identity Disorder: C. Inability to recall important personal information that is too extensive to be explained by ordinary forgetfulness.		____	____
SCID-D items supporting Criterion C: 1) Significant amnesia for personal information.	1–17	____	____

Dissociative Identity Disorder

Diagnostic Work Sheet

	SCID-D items	Yes	No
DSM-IV Criterion D for Dissociative Identity Disorder:			
D. The disturbance is not due to the direct physiological effects of a substance (e.g., blackouts or chaotic behavior during Alcohol Intoxication) or a general medical condition (e.g., complex partial seizures). **Note:** In children, the symptoms are not attributable to imaginary playmates or other fantasy play.		____	____
SCID-D items supporting Criterion D:			
1) The dissociative symptoms were not initiated and/or maintained exclusively by drugs or alcohol.	24–28, 31–35, 72–76, 95–99	____	____

SCID-D inclusion criteria for Dissociative Identity Disorder based on severity and clinical significance of symptoms:
The following constellation of clinically significant dissociative symptoms is present:

	Symptom	Severity rating	Yes	No
i)	Amnesia	Moderate to Severe	____	____
ii)	Depersonalization Derealization	Moderate to Severe in at least one of these symptoms	____	____
iii)	Identity confusion*	Moderate to Severe	____	____
iv)	Identity alteration	Moderate to Severe	____	____

***Note:** Subjects with severe amnesia may deny awareness of identity confusion.

(See SCID-D Severity Rating Definitions for further information.)

Prepared for use in conjunction with Steinberg M: *Interviewer's Guide to the Structured Clinical Interview for DSM-IV Dissociative Disorders* (SCID-D), Revised. Washington, DC, American Psychiatric Press, 1994.

Exclusion Criteria for Dissociative Identity Disorder

Diagnostic Work Sheet

	SCID-D items	Yes	No
SCID-D exclusion criteria for Dissociative Identity Disorder: The presence of any of the following rules out the diagnosis of Dissociative Identity Disorder:			
A. Exclusion criteria regarding context and content of symptoms			
1) The dissociative symptoms were initiated and/or maintained exclusively by drugs, alcohol, or medical illness.	24–28, 31–35, 72–76, 95–99	____	____
2) The following criteria strongly suggest a diagnosis of Schizophrenia or Delusional (paranoid) Disorder:			
a) Hallucinations other than the voices of the different personalities conversing with each other.		____	____
b) Bizarre, paranoid, or other delusions that do not involve the individual's perceptions, feelings, or reactions to the other personalities, e.g., paranoid delusions such as "The CIA is out to get me."		____	____
c) Thinking characterized by incoherence or marked loosening of associations.		____	____
d) Catatonic behavior.		____	____
e) Chronic flat affect.		____	____
f) The dissociative symptoms occurred exclusively during the course of a psychotic disturbance or were brief in duration relative to the duration of psychotic symptoms.		____	____
g) The identity disturbance is associated only with an imagined identity of a fictional character, famous person, deity, or other delusional identity, e.g., belief that he/she is Jesus Christ.		____	____

Subject's initials ______________ Date ____________

Interviewer ________________

Depersonalization Disorder

Diagnostic Work Sheet

	SCID-D items	Yes	No
DSM-IV Criterion A for Depersonalization Disorder:			
A. Persistent or recurrent experiences of feeling detached from, and as if one is an outside observer of, one's mental processes or body (e.g., feeling like one is in a dream).		___	___
SCID-D items supporting Criterion A:			
1) Persistent or recurrent depersonalization episodes as indicated by one of the following:			
a) an experience of observing one's self, as if one is an outside observer of one's body	38, 47	___	___
b) a sensation of self-estrangement or unreality, which may include the feeling that one's extremities have changed in size (DSM-III-R)	40, 41, 44, 49	___	___
c) an experience of feeling detached from one's behavior or body as if in a dream	38, 43, 46, 47, 50–53	___	___
DSM-IV Criterion B for Depersonalization Disorder:			
B. During the depersonalization experience, reality testing remains intact.		___	___
SCID-D criteria supporting Criterion B:			
1) During the depersonalization episode, the subject was otherwise in touch with reality.	38–53	___	___

Depersonalization Disorder
Diagnostic Work Sheet

	SCID-D items	Yes	No
DSM-IV Criterion C for Depersonalization Disorder:			
C. The depersonalization causes marked distress or significant impairment in social or occupational functioning.		____	____
SCID-D items supporting Criterion C: The presence of all of the following:			
1) Recurrent or persistent episodes of depersonalization.	39, 45, 48, 55, 56	____	____
2) The depersonalization episodes cause marked distress.	65	____	____
3) The depersonalization episodes cause impairment in social or occupational functioning.	63	____	____
DSM-IV Criterion D for Depersonalization Disorder:			
D. The depersonalization experience does not occur exclusively during the course of another mental disorder, such as Schizophrenia, Panic Disorder, Acute Stress Disorder, or another Dissociative Disorder, and is not due to the direct physiological effects of a substance (e.g., a drug of abuse, a medication) or a general medical condition (e.g., temporal lobe epilepsy).		____	____
SCID-D items supporting Criterion D: The presence of all of the following:			
1) The depersonalization episode is not a symptom of another disorder, such as Schizophrenia or Panic Disorder.	57–71	____	____
2) The depersonalization episode is not a symptom of temporal lobe epilepsy or other medical condition.	72–76	____	____
3) The depersonalization episode is not initiated and/or maintained exclusively by drugs or alcohol.	72–76	____	____
4) The depersonalization is not a symptom of Dissociative Identity Disorder. (See Dissociative Identity Disorder Diagnostic Work Sheet.)		____	____

Depersonalization Disorder

Diagnostic Work Sheet

	SCID-D items	Yes	No
SCID-D inclusion criteria for Depersonalization Disorder based on severity and clinical significance of symptoms: The following constellation of clinically significant symptoms is present:			

	Symptom	Severity rating	Yes	No
i)	Amnesia	Absent to Moderate	____	____
ii)	Depersonalization	Severe	____	____
iii)	Derealization*	Absent to Moderate	____	____
iv)	Identity confusion*	Absent to Mild	____	____
v)	Identity alteration	Absent to Mild	____	____

***Note:** In patients with Depersonalization Disorder, significant derealization and identity confusion occur only in conjunction with depersonalization.

(See SCID-D Severity Rating Definitions for further information.)

Exclusion Criteria for Depersonalization Disorder

Diagnostic Work Sheet

	SCID-D items	Yes	No
SCID-D exclusion criteria for Depersonalization Disorder: The presence of any of the following rules out the diagnosis of Depersonalization Disorder:			
A. Exclusion criteria regarding context and content of symptoms			
1) The depersonalization symptoms were initiated and/or maintained exclusively by drugs, alcohol, medical illness, or seizure disorder.	72–76	____	____
2) The following criteria strongly suggest a diagnosis of Schizophrenia or a psychotic disorder:			
a) Any bizarre or paranoid delusions ("Delusions are deemed bizarre if they are clearly implausible and not understandable and do not derive from ordinary life experiences" [DSM-IV, p. 275]).		____	____
b) Thinking characterized by incoherence or marked loosening of associations.		____	____
c) The depersonalization episodes occurred exclusively during the course of a psychotic illness or only in association with psychotic symptoms.	67	____	____
3) The subject has Dissociative Identity Disorder. The existence of Dissociative Identity Disorder subsumes all of the Dissociative Disorders. If Dissociative Identity Disorder is suspected, the interviewer should consult the Dissociative Identity Disorder Diagnostic Work Sheet to rule out that diagnosis.		____	____

Prepared for use in conjunction with Steinberg M: *Interviewer's Guide to the Structured Clinical Interview for DSM-IV Dissociative Disorders* (SCID-D), Revised. Washington, DC, American Psychiatric Press, 1994.

Subject's initials ______________ Date ____________

Interviewer ________________

Dissociative Disorder Not Otherwise Specified (DDNOS)

Diagnostic Work Sheet

	SCID-D items	Yes	No
DSM-IV definition: Disorders in which the predominant feature is a dissociative symptom (i.e., a disruption in the usually integrative functions of consciousness, memory, identity, or perception of the environment) that does not meet the criteria for any specific Dissociative Disorder.		____	____

Explanation: Because DDNOS is a residual category, DSM-IV describes various forms. The DDNOS Diagnostic Work Sheet deals with the two most common categories of DDNOS. The first category (DSM-IV Example 1) involves cases very similar to Dissociative Identity Disorder (Multiple Personality Disorder), but lacking an essential feature of Dissociative Identity Disorder. Example 1A characterizes individuals with personality states that take control of behavior and thought but are not sufficiently distinct for a diagnosis of Dissociative Identity Disorder. Example 1B characterizes individuals who have distinct and volitional personality states but lack amnesia for important personal information. The second major category of DDNOS (DSM-IV Example 2) simply involves cases of derealization unaccompanied by depersonalization. The other types of DDNOS are less common and have not been included in the Diagnostic Work Sheet. Information about dissociative symptoms from the SCID-D may nevertheless be used to assess these other types of DDNOS.

DDNOS

Diagnostic Work Sheet

DDNOS Categories to follow:

DSM-IV Example 1—Cases similar to Dissociative Identity Disorder:

1A. Clinical presentations similar to Dissociative Identity Disorder that fail to meet full criteria for this disorder. Examples include presentations in which a) there are not two or more distinct personality states, or b) amnesia for important personal information does not occur.
[IF YES: Go to DDNOS Example 1A Diagnostic Work Sheet]

1B. Cases similar to Dissociative Identity Disorder but in which there is no amnesia for important personal information.
[IF YES: Go to DDNOS Example 1B Diagnostic Work Sheet]

DSM-IV Example 2—Cases of derealization without depersonalization in adults
[IF YES: Go to DDNOS Example 2 Diagnostic Work Sheet]

Subject's initials ______________ Date ___________

Interviewer ________________

DDNOS

Example 1A Diagnostic Work Sheet

	SCID-D items	Yes	No
DSM-IV Example 1A: Clinical presentations similar to Dissociative Identity Disorder that fail to meet full criteria for this disorder. Examples include presentations in which a) there are not two or more distinct personality states, or b) amnesia for important personal information does not occur.		____	____
SCID-D items supporting Example 1A: All of the following must be present:			
1) Recurrent or persistent feeling that two or more identities exist within him/herself, as indicated by at least one of the following:			
a) recurrent or persistent feeling that he/she is two different people, one going through the motions of life and the other observing	46, 47	____	____
b) recurrent or persistent feeling that he/she acts as if he/she were a different person or he/she is told by others that he/she seems like a different person	114, 116	____	____
c) use of different names, or being called by others by different names (not nicknames or an alias used only to facilitate illegal activity)	118, 120	____	____
2) None of the personality states is sufficiently distinct to meet the full criteria of Dissociative Identity Disorder.	(see follow-up sections)	____	____
3) At least two of these personalities or personality states recurrently take control of the person's behavior, as indicated by one of the following:			
a) history of alterations in his/her demeanor, as if he/she were two different people	134, 135	____	____

DDNOS Example 1A

Diagnostic Work Sheet

	SCID-D items	Yes	No
b) alterations in his/her speech (i.e., vocabulary, accents), and/or behavior that is not under his/her control	(see follow-up sections)	____	____
c) intra-interview manifestations of alterations in subject's identity, as indicated by at least one of the following:			
1. dramatic alterations in subject's demeanor during interview	259	____	____
2. alterations in subject's identity	260	____	____
3. spontaneous age regression	261	____	____
4) Associated features of a Dissociative Disorder as indicated by at least two of the following:			
a) recurrent amnestic episodes	1–7, 17	____	____
b) recurrent or persistent depersonalization	38–47	____	____
c) recurrent or persistent derealization	79–84	____	____
d) several depersonalization episodes that (one of the following):			
1. produce impairment in social or occupational functioning	63	____	____
2. are not precipitated by stressful events	64	____	____
3. are prolonged (lasting over 4 hours)	55	____	____
e) rapid fluctuations in symptoms, mood, or level of functioning	134–135	____	____
5) Intra-interview cues of alter personalities or of a Dissociative Disorder, as indicated by at least one of the following:			
a) marked alterations in subject's demeanor	259	____	____
b) alterations in subject's identity	260	____	____
c) spontaneous age regression	261	____	____
d) intra-interview amnesia	265	____	____
e) subject refers to him/herself in the third person	263	____	____
f) significant emotional response to SCID-D questions	270	____	____
g) trancelike appearance	272	____	____

DDNOS EXAMPLE 1A

Diagnostic Work Sheet

	SCID-D items	Yes	No
SCID-D inclusion criteria for DDNOS, Example 1A, based on severity and clinical significance of symptoms: The following constellation of clinically significant dissociative symptoms is present:			

	Symptom	Severity rating		Yes	No
i)	Amnesia	Absent to Severe		____	____
ii)	Depersonalization	Absent to Severe		____	____
iii)	Derealization	Absent to Severe		____	____
iv)	Identity confusion	Mild to Severe		____	____
v)	Identity alteration	Moderate to Severe		____	____

(See SCID-D Severity Rating Definitions for further information.)

Subject's initials ______________ Date ___________
Interviewer ________________

DDNOS

Example 1B Diagnostic Work Sheet

	SCID-D items	Yes	No
DSM-IV Example 1B: Cases similar to Dissociative Identity Disorder but in which there is no amnesia for important personal information.			
SCID-D items supporting Example 1B: All of the following must be present:			
1) Recurrent or persistent feeling that two or more people exist within him/herself, as indicated by at least one of the following:			
a) recurrent or persistent feeling that he/she is two different people, one going through the motions of life and the other observing	46, 47	____	____
b) recurrent or persistent feeling that he/she acts as if he/she were a different person or he/she is told by others that he/she seems like a different person	114, 116	____	____
c) use of different names, or being called by others by different names (not nicknames or an alias used only to facilitate illegal activity)	118, 120	____	____
2) Persistent manifestations of the presence of different personalities, as indicated by at least four of the following:			
a) ongoing dialogues between the two different people	138–145	____	____
b) sudden acting or feeling that the different people inside of him/her take control of his/her behavior or speech	(see follow-up sections)	____	____
c) characteristic visual image that is associated with the other person, distinct from subject	(see follow-up sections)	____	____
d) characteristic age associated with the different people inside of him/her	(see follow-up sections)	____	____

DDNOS Example 1B

Diagnostic Work Sheet

	SCID-D items	Yes	No
e) feeling that the different people inside of him/her have different memories, behaviors, and feelings	(see follow-up sections)	____	____
f) feeling that the different people inside of him/her are separate from his/her personality and have lives of their own	(see follow-up sections)	____	____
3) The personality states assume control of behavior and thought.	(see follow-up sections)	____	____
4) Associated features of a Dissociative Disorder as indicated by at least two of the following:			
a) recurrent amnestic episodes	1–7, 17	____	____
b) recurrent or persistent depersonalization	38–47	____	____
c) recurrent or persistent derealization	79–84	____	____
d) several depersonalization episodes that (one of the following):			
1. produce impairment in social or occupational functioning	63	____	____
2. are not precipitated by stressful events	64	____	____
3. are prolonged (lasting over 4 hours)	55	____	____
e) rapid fluctuations in symptoms, mood, or level of functioning	134, 135	____	____
5) Intra-interview cues of alter personalities or of a Dissociative Disorder, as indicated by at least two of the following:			
a) intra-interview amnesia	265	____	____
b) subject refers to him/herself in the third person	263	____	____
c) significant emotional response to SCID-D questions	270	____	____
d) trancelike appearance	272	____	____
6) Amnesia for important personal information does not occur.	1–17	____	____

DDNOS EXAMPLE 1B

Diagnostic Work Sheet

	SCID-D items	Yes	No

SCID-D inclusion criteria for DDNOS Example 1B,
based on severity and clinical significance of symptoms:
The following constellation of clinically significant dissociative symptoms are present:

	Symptom	Severity rating	Yes	No
i)	Amnesia	Absent to Mild	_____	_____
ii)	Depersonalization	Absent to Severe	_____	_____
iii)	Derealization	Absent to Severe	_____	_____
iv)	Identity confusion	Moderate to Severe	_____	_____
v)	Identity Alteration	Moderate to Severe	_____	_____

(See SCID-D Severity Rating Definitions for further information.)

Subject's initials ______________ Date ___________
Interviewer ________________

DDNOS

Example 2 Diagnostic Work Sheet

	SCID-D items	Yes	No
DSM-IV Example 2: Derealization unaccompanied by depersonalization in adults.			
SCID-D items supporting Example 2: All of the following must be present:			
1) Recurrent or persistent episodes of derealization (without depersonalization) as indicated by at least one of the following:			
a) feeling that his/her environment is unreal	79–85	____	____
b) feeling that familiar surroundings or people he/she knows seem unfamiliar or unreal	79–85	____	____
2) The derealization episode is the predominant disturbance. (See Severity Rating Definitions.)	79–85 (all of SCID-D)	____	____
3) Absence of depersonalization	38–48	____	____

SCID-D inclusion criteria for DDNOS, Example 2, based on severity and clinical significance of symptoms:
The following constellation of clinically significant dissociative symptoms must be present:

	Symptom	Severity rating	Yes	No
i)	Amnesia	Absent to Mild	____	____
ii)	Depersonalization	Absent	____	____
iii)	Derealization	Moderate to Severe	____	____
iv)	Identity confusion	Absent to Mild	____	____
v)	Identity alteration	Absent to Mild	____	____

(See SCID-D Severity Rating Definitions for further information.)

Exclusion Criteria for DDNOS, DSM-IV Examples 1 (A & B) and 2

Diagnostic Work Sheet

	SCID-D items	Yes	No
SCID-D exclusion criteria for DDNOS: The presence of any of the following rules out the diagnosis of DDNOS, DSM-IV Examples 1 (A & B) and 2:			
A. Exclusion criteria regarding context and content of symptoms			
1) The following criteria strongly suggest a diagnosis of a *specific* Dissociative Disorder (i.e., one of the first four in DSM-IV) or organic mental syndrome and exclude the diagnosis of DDNOS:			
a) The dissociative symptoms were initiated and/or maintained exclusively by drugs, alcohol, or medical illness	24–28, 31–35, 72–76, 95–99	____	____
b) The dissociative symptoms are in the context of a specific Dissociative Disorder. (See other Diagnostic Work Sheets.)		____	____
2) The following criteria strongly suggest a diagnosis of Schizophrenia or Delusional (paranoid) Disorder and exclude the diagnosis of DDNOS:			
a) Hallucinations other than the voices of the different personalities conversing with each other.		____	____
b) Bizarre, paranoid, or other delusions that do not involve the individual's perceptions, feelings, or reactions to the other personalities, i.e., paranoid delusions such as "The CIA is out to get me."		____	____
c) Thinking characterized by incoherence or marked loosening of associations.		____	____
d) Catatonic behavior.		____	____
e) Chronic flat affect.		____	____
f) The dissociative symptoms occurred exclusively during the course of a psychotic disturbance or were brief in duration relative to the duration of psychotic symptoms.		____	____

Subject's initials ______________ Date ___________

Interviewer ________________

Dissociative Trance Disorder

Diagnostic Work Sheet

> **Note:** Dissociative Trance Disorder is categorized as a subtype of Dissociative Disorder Not Otherwise Specified in DSM-IV. The criteria below are taken from Appendix B, "Criteria Sets and Axes Provided for Further Study," of DSM-IV. The SCID-D can be used by clinicians and researchers for the evaluation of Dissociative Trance Disorder. See also the SCID-D "Feeling of Possession" follow-up section.

	SCID-D items	Yes	No
DSM-IV Research Criterion A for Dissociative Trance Disorder:		____	____

A. Either 1) or 2):

1) Trance, i.e., temporary marked alteration in the state of consciousness or loss of customary sense of personal identity without replacement by an alternate identity, associated with at least one of the following:

   a) narrowing of awareness of immediate surroundings, or unusually narrow and selective focusing on environmental stimuli
   b) stereotyped behaviors or movements that are experienced as being beyond one's control

2) Possession trance, a single or episodic alteration in the state of consciousness characterized by the replacement of customary sense of personal identity by a new identity. This is attributed to the influence of a spirit, power, deity, or other person, as evidenced by one (or more) of the following:

   a) stereotyped and culturally determined behaviors or movements that are experienced as being controlled by the possessing agent
   b) full or partial amnesia for the event

Dissociative Trance Disorder

Diagnostic Work Sheet

	SCID-D items	Yes	No
SCID-D items supporting Criterion A (at least one of the following):			
1) Episodes of trance as indicated by one of the following:			
a) loss of customary sense of personal identity or confusion regarding one's identity	11–15, 101–105	____	____
b) narrowing of awareness of surroundings or other manifestations of derealization	101–105, 79–84, 272	____	____
c) stereotyped behaviors or movements that are experienced as being beyond one's control	50–53, 170–180, 245–258	____	____
2) Episodes of possession, as evidenced by at least one of the following:			
a) conviction that the individual has been taken over by a spirit, power, deity, or other person	124–125, 245–258	____	____
b) amnesia for the event	1–15	____	____
DSM-IV Research Criterion B for Dissociative Trance Disorder:			
B. The trance or possession trance state is not accepted as a normal part of a collective cultural or religious practice.		____	____
SCID-D criteria supporting Criterion B:			
1) The trance or possession state is not a normal part of a broadly accepted collective cultural or religious practice.	256	____	____
DSM-IV Research Criterion C for Dissociative Trance Disorder:			
C. The trance or possession trance state causes clinically significant distress or impairment in social, occupational, or other important areas of functioning.		____	____
SCID-D items supporting Criterion C: The presence of one of the following:			
1) The trance or possession state causes impairment in social or occupational functioning.	256a	____	____
2) The possession state causes marked distress.	256b	____	____

Dissociative Trance Disorder

Diagnostic Work Sheet

	SCID-D items	Yes	No
DSM-IV Research Criterion D for Dissociative Trance Disorder:			
D. The trance or possession trance state does not occur exclusively during the course of a Psychotic Disorder (including Mood Disorder With Psychotic Features and Brief Psychotic Disorder) or Dissociative Identity Disorder and is not due to the direct physiological effects of a substance or a general medical condition.	all of SCID-D	____	____
SCID-D items supporting Criterion D: The presence of one of the following:			
1) The trance or possession state does not occur during the course of a psychotic disorder, Dissociative Identity Disorder, Substance Abuse Disorder, or general medical condition.	all of SCID-D	____	____

SCID-D inclusion criteria for Dissociative Trance Disorder based on severity and clinical significance of symptoms:
The following constellation of clinically significant symptoms is present:*

	Symptom	Severity rating	Yes	No
i)	Amnesia	Mild to Severe	____	____
ii)	Depersonalization	Moderate to Severe	____	____
iii)	Derealization	Mild to Severe	____	____
iv)	Identity confusion	Moderate to Severe	____	____
v)	Identity alteration	Moderate to Severe	____	____

(See SCID-D Severity Rating Definitions for further information.)

Prepared for use in conjunction with Steinberg M: *Interviewer's Guide to the Structured Clinical Interview for DSM-IV Dissociative Disorders* (SCID-D), Revised. Washington, DC, American Psychiatric Press, 1994.

Exclusion Criteria for Dissociative Trance Disorder

Diagnostic Work Sheet

	SCID-D items	Yes	No
SCID-D exclusion criteria for Dissociative Trance Disorder: The presence of any of the following rules out the diagnosis of Dissociative Trance Disorder:			
A. Exclusion criteria regarding context and content of symptoms			
1) The trance or possession symptoms were initiated and/or maintained exclusively by drugs, alcohol, medical illness, or seizure disorder.		____	____
2) The following criteria strongly suggest a diagnosis of Schizophrenia or Delusional (paranoid) Disorder:			
a) Hallucinations other than the voices or images of the possessing agent(s).		____	____
b) Bizarre, paranoid, or other delusions that do not involve the individual's perceptions, feelings, or reactions to the possessing agent(s).		____	____
c) The dissociative symptoms occurred exclusively during the course of a psychotic disturbance or were brief in duration relative to the duration of psychotic symptoms.		____	____
3) The trance or possession episodes only occur secondary to a medical condition.		____	____
4) The subject has Dissociative Identity. The existence of Dissociative Identity Disorder subsumes all of the Dissociative Disorders. If Dissociative Identity Disorder is suspected, the interviewer should consult the Dissociative Identity Disorder Diagnostic Work Sheet to rule out that diagnosis.		____	____

Subject's initials ______________ Date ___________
Interviewer _________________

Acute Stress Disorder

Diagnostic Work Sheet

Note: Acute Stress Disorder is a new category introduced in the Anxiety Disorders section of DSM-IV. The criteria for this disorder are included on the Diagnostic Work Sheet that follows. Note that Criterion B specifies that the person manifest at least three of five dissociative symptoms. Because these symptoms are assessed by the SCID-D, clinicians can use the instrument to diagnose the presence of Acute Stress Disorder.

	SCID-D items	Yes	No
DSM-IV Criterion A for Acute Stress Disorder:		____	____
A. The person has been exposed to a traumatic event in which both of the following were present:			
1) The person experienced, witnessed, or was confronted with an event or events that involved actual or threatened death or serious injury or a threat to the physical integrity of self or others.			
2) The person's response involved intense fear, helplessness, or horror.			
SCID-D items supporting Criterion A:			
1) Traumatic experience involving actual or threatened death or physical injury.	psychiatric history	____	____
2) Spontaneous reports of trauma.	all of SCID-D	____	____
3) The person's response involved intense fear, helplessness, and/or horror.	psychiatric history	____	____

ACUTE STRESS DISORDER

Diagnostic Work Sheet

	SCID-D items	Yes	No
DSM-IV Criterion B for Acute Stress Disorder (Acute Anxiety and Dissociative Disorder):		____	____

B. Either while experiencing or after experiencing the distressing event, the individual has three (or more) of the following dissociative symptoms:

1) a subjective sense of numbing, detachment, or absence of emotional responsiveness
2) a reduction in awareness of his or her surroundings (e.g., "being in a daze")
3) derealization
4) depersonalization
5) dissociative amnesia (i.e., inability to recall an important aspect of the trauma)

SCID-D items supporting Criterion B:
The following dissociative symptoms occurred during or after the traumatic experience (three [or more] of the following):

	SCID-D items	Yes	No
1) feeling numb or having difficulty experiencing emotion	psychiatric history, 38–53	____	____
2) stupor, feeling dazed, or feeling out of touch with reality	psychiatric history, 38–53, 79–84, 272	____	____
3) experiencing the environment as unreal	psychiatric history, 79–84	____	____
4) feeling unreal or detached from oneself	psychiatric history, 38–53	____	____
5) feeling detached or estranged from others	psychiatric history, 79–84, 267	____	____
6) amnesia for events associated with the traumatic experience	psychiatric history, 1–15, 265	____	____

Acute Stress Disorder

Diagnostic Work Sheet

	SCID-D items	Yes	No
DSM-IV Criterion C for Acute Stress Disorder C. The traumatic event is persistently reexperienced in at least one of the following ways: recurrent images, thoughts, dreams, illusions, flashback episodes, or a sense of reliving the experience; or distress on exposure to reminders of the traumatic event.		____	____
SCID-D items supporting Criterion C: Either 1 or 2 must be present:			
1) reliving the trauma (e.g., flashbacks)	psychiatric history, 136, 223–233	____	____
2) distress when reminded of traumatic event(s)	psychiatric history, 223–233	____	____
DSM-IV Criterion D for Acute Stress Disorder: D. Marked avoidance of stimuli that arouse recollections of the trauma (e.g., thoughts, feelings, conversations, activities, places, people).		____	____
SCID-D items supporting Criterion D: Avoidance of situations that remind patient of the trauma	psychiatric history	____	____
DSM-IV Criterion E for Acute Stress Disorder: E. Marked symptoms of anxiety or increased arousal (e.g., difficulty sleeping, irritability, poor concentration, hypervigilance, exaggerated startle response, motor restlessness).		____	____
SCID-D items supporting Criterion E: At least two of the following anxiety symptoms are present:			
1) difficulty sleeping	psychiatric history	____	____
2) irritability	psychiatric history	____	____
3) poor concentration	psychiatric history	____	____

ACUTE STRESS DISORDER
Diagnostic Work Sheet

	SCID-D items	Yes	No
4) hypervigilance	psychiatric history	____	____
5) exaggerated startle response	psychiatric history	____	____
6) motor restlessness	psychiatric history	____	____

		Yes	No
DSM-IV Criterion F for Acute Stress Disorder: F. The disturbance causes clinically significant distress or impairment in social, occupational, or other important areas of functioning or impairs the individual's ability to pursue some necessary task, such as obtaining necessary assistance or mobilizing personal resources by telling family members about the traumatic experience.		____	____
SCID-D items supporting Criterion F:			
1) The symptoms cause interference in social or occupational functioning.	psychiatric history, entire interview	____	____
2) The symptoms cause marked distress or discomfort.	psychiatric history, entire interview	____	____

		Yes	No
DSM-IV Criterion G for Acute Stress Disorder: G. The disturbance lasts for a minimum of 2 days and a maximum of 4 weeks and occurs within 4 weeks of the traumatic event.		____	____
SCID-D items supporting Criterion G:			
The disturbance lasts more than 2 days and less than 4 weeks.	psychiatric history	____	____

ACUTE STRESS DISORDER
Diagnostic Work Sheet

	SCID-D items	Yes	No
DSM-IV Criterion H for Acute Stress Disorder: H. The disturbance is not due to the direct physiological effects of a substance (e.g., a drug of abuse, a medication) or a general medical condition, is not better accounted for by Brief Psychotic Disorder, and is not merely an exacerbation of a preexisting Axis I or Axis II disorder. of 4 weeks and occurs within 4 weeks of the traumatic event.		____	____
SCID-D items supporting Criterion H:			
1) The disturbance is not induced by alcohol or drugs.	psychiatric history, 24–28, 31–35, 72–76, 132–133	____	____
2) The disturbance is not due to a general medical condition.	psychiatric history	____	____
3) The disturbance is not due to an exacerbation of a preexisting Axis I or Axis II disorder.	psychiatric history	____	____

EXCLUSION CRITERIA FOR ACUTE STRESS DISORDER
Diagnostic Work Sheet

	SCID-D items	Yes	No
SCID-D exclusion criteria for Acute Stress Disorder: The presence of any of the following rules out the diagnosis of Acute Stress Disorder:			
A. Exclusion criteria regarding context and content of symptoms			
1) The dissociative symptoms were initiated and/or maintained exclusively by drugs, alcohol, or seizure disorder.		____	____
2) The following criteria strongly suggest a diagnosis of Schizophrenia or Delusional (paranoid) Disorder:			
a) the presence of prominent hallucinations or bizarre delusions		____	____
b) thinking characterized by incoherence or marked loosening of associations		____	____
3) The dissociative episodes only occur secondary to a medical condition.		____	____
4) The subject has Dissociative Identity Disorder. The existence of Dissociative Identity Disorder subsumes all of the Dissociative Disorders. If Dissociative Identity Disorder is suspected, the interviewer should consult the Dissociative Identity Disorder Diagnostic Work Sheet to rule out that diagnosis.		____	____

APPENDIX 3

Depersonalization Section of Sample SCID-D Interview

Depersonalization

Past Symptoms/Current Symptoms

Some people have had experiences that feel very real to them but are very hard to explain to other people. Now, I am going to ask you about some of these experiences.

38. Have you ever felt that you were watching yourself from a point outside of your body, as if you were seeing yourself from a distance (or watching a movie of yourself)?

IF YES: What is that experience like?
DESCRIBE:

2 ways:
1) "traveling inside"
2) "sitting next to myself"

Depersonalization ? N (Y) I

"An alteration in the perception or experience of the self so that one feels detached from, and as if one is an outside observer of, one's mental processes or body (e.g., feeling like one is in a dream)" (DSM-IV, p. 766).

"Patients feel that their point of conscious 'I-ness' is outside their bodies, commonly a few feet overhead, from where they actually observe themselves as if they were a totally other person" (Nemiah 1989, p. 1042).

39. How often have you had that experience?
(Rate most frequent period.)

few times/week

Frequency of Depersonalization

- ❐ unclear
- ❐ rarely (up to 4 isolated episodes)
- ❐ occasionally (up to 4 episodes per year)
- ❐ frequently (5 episodes or more per year)
- ❐ monthly episodes (up to 3 per month)
- ☑ daily or weekly episodes (4 or more per month)

40. Have you ever had the feeling that you were a stranger to yourself? ? N (Y) I

IF YES: What is that experience like?
(How often does that occur?)

DESCRIBE:
"Those are not my hands."
"That's not my face."
"It's scary."

? = inadequate information N = no Y = yes I = inconsistent information

41. Have you ever felt as if a part of your body or your whole being was foreign to you? ? N (Y) I

IF YES: What is that experience like? (How often does that occur?) DESCRIBE: "hands"

42. Have you ever had the feeling that part of your body was disconnected (detached) from the rest of your body? ? N (Y) I

IF YES: What is that experience like? (How often does that occur?) DESCRIBE: "My head is detached from the rest of my body."

43. Have you ever felt as if part of your body or your whole body disappeared? ? (N) Y I

(Have you ever felt that you were fading away?)

IF YES: What is that experience like? (How often does that occur?) DESCRIBE:

44. Have you ever felt as if parts of your body or your whole being was unreal? ? N (Y) I

IF YES: What is that experience like? DESCRIBE: "My hands are not real."

45. How often have you had that experience?
(Rate most frequent period.)

1–2x/week

Frequency of Depersonalization
- ❒ unclear
- ❒ rarely (up to 4 isolated episodes)
- ❒ occasionally (up to 4 episodes per year)
- ❒ frequently (5 episodes or more per year)
- ❒ monthly episodes (up to 3 per month)
- ☑ daily or weekly episodes (4 or more per month)

46. Have you ever felt that you were going through the motions of living but that the real you was far away from what was happening to you? ? N (Y) I

(Have you ever felt that you were going through the motions of participating in life, but you really felt detached from your behavior?) (Have you ever felt that you were participating in life, but you felt as if you were living in a dream?)

? = inadequate information N = no Y = yes I = inconsistent information

IF YES: What is that experience like? (How often does that occur?)

DESCRIBE: "My body's just moving and I'm not really there."

? N (Y) I

47. Have you ever felt as if you were two different people, one person going through the motions of life and the other observing quietly?

IF YES: What is that experience like?

DESCRIBE: "I go inside... I retreat."

48. How often does that occur?
(Rate most frequent period.)

1–2x/week

Frequency of Depersonalization

- ❒ unclear
- ❒ rarely (up to 4 isolated episodes)
- ❒ occasionally (up to 4 episodes per year)
- ❒ frequently (5 episodes or more per year)
- ❒ monthly episodes (up to 3 per month)
- ☑ daily or weekly episodes (4 or more per month)

*49. Have you ever felt that your arms or legs were bigger or smaller than usual or were changing in size?

? N (Y) I

IF YES: When you felt that your ______ were ______ than usual, what was that experience like? "I felt very little."

*50. Have you ever heard yourself talking and felt that you were not the one choosing the words?

DESCRIBE: "I said something that I didn't mean and that was very offensive."

? N (Y) I

(Have you ever felt as if words seem to flow from your mouth as if they were not in your control?)

In depersonalization, "a sensation of lacking control of one's actions, including speech," is often present (DSM-IV, p. 488).

IF YES: What is that experience like? (How often does that occur?)

DESCRIBE:

? = inadequate information N = no Y = yes I = inconsistent information

*51. Have you ever felt as if your behavior was not in your control? ? N (Y) I

IF YES: What is that experience like? (How often does that occur?)

DESCRIBE: "Buying things I didn't plan to buy"

*52. Have you ever felt as if your emotions were not in your control? ? N (Y) I

IF YES: What is that experience like? (How often does that occur?)

DESCRIBE:

*53. Have you ever felt as if you were a puppet under someone else's control? ? N (Y) I

IF YES: What is that experience like?

DESCRIBE: "I'm being played out."

IF SUBJECT DESCRIBED A DEPERSONALIZATION EPISODE, CONTINUE WITH #54.
IF NO DEPERSONALIZATION, GO TO PAGE 25 (DEREALIZATION SECTION).

54.

Rate Overall Frequency of Most Severe Depersonalization

- ☐ unclear
- ☐ rarely (up to 4 isolated episodes)
- ☐ occasionally (up to 4 episodes per year)
- ☐ frequently (5 episodes or more per year)
- ☐ monthly episodes (up to 3 per month)
- ☑ daily or weekly episodes (4 or more per month)

55. What is the longest period of time that ______ (endorsed symptoms of depersonalization) have ever lasted?

at least days

- ☑ time period is unclear
- ☐ minutes
- ☐ less than 4 hours
- ☐ less than 24 hours
- ☐ less than 1 week
- ☐ less than 1 month
- ☐ 1 month or longer

? = inadequate information N = no Y = yes I = inconsistent information

*56. Does each experience of

____
(endorsed symptoms of depersonalization)

last for about the same amount of time?

(Do some experiences of

____
(endorsed symptoms of depersonalization)

take much more or much less time?)

Pattern of Depersonalization

- ❒ unclear
- ❒ variable frequency
- ❒ constant

*57. Does the experience of

____
(endorsed symptoms of depersonalization)

begin suddenly or gradually?

- ❒ onset is unclear
- ❒ onset is usually sudden
- ❒ onset varies
- ❒ onset is usually gradual

58.

Depersonalization Disorder Criterion A ? N (Y) I

A. Persistent or recurrent experiences of feeling detached from, and as if one is an outside observer of, one's mental processes or body (e.g., feeling like one is in a dream).

59.

Depersonalization Disorder Criterion B ? N (Y) I

B. During the depersonalization experience, reality testing remains intact.

*60. How old were you when you first experienced ______________________

______________? (endorsed symptoms of depersonalization)

Age at Onset of Depersonalization

- ❒ age at onset is unclear
- ☑ during early childhood (up to age 6)
- ❒ during childhood (ages 7–12)
- ❒ during adolescence (ages 13–19)
- ❒ young adult (ages 20–30)
- ❒ adult (over age 31)

? = inadequate information N = no Y = yes I = inconsistent information

*61. How old were you the last time that you experienced ________________________ ? (endorsed symptoms of depersonalization)

- ❒ unclear
- ❒ during early childhood (up to age 6)
- ❒ during childhood (ages 7–12)
- ❒ during adolescence (ages 13–19)
- ❒ young adult (ages 20–30)
- ❒ adult (over age 31)

*62.

Rate Most Recent Episode

- ❒ unclear
- ❒ occurred prior to past year
- ❒ occurred during past year
- ❒ occurred during past month

63. When you experience ________________________, (endorsed symptoms of depersonalization) **does it ever interfere with your social relationships or affect your ability to work?**

? N (Y) I

IF YES: How does it interfere with your social relationships? How does it interfere with your ability to work?

DESCRIBE: Behaves inappropriately

64. Is the experience of ________________________ (endorsed symptoms of depersonalization) **associated with stress?**

- ❒ unclear
- ❒ not associated with stress
- ☑ sometimes associated with stress
- ❒ usually associated with stress

65. When you experience ________________________, (endorsed symptoms of depersonalization) **does this cause you discomfort or distress?**

- ❒ unclear
- ☑ does not cause distress (may be comforting)
- ❒ sometimes causes distress
- ❒ usually causes distress

66.

Depersonalization Disorder Criterion C ? N (Y) I

C. The depersonalization causes clinically significant distress or impairment in social, occupational, or other important areas of functioning.

IF SUBJECT MEETS DEPERSONALIZATION CRITERIA, CONTINUE WITH #67.

? = inadequate information N = no Y = yes I = inconsistent information

IF SUBJECT DOES NOT MEET DEPERSONALIZATION CRITERIA, GO TO PAGE 25 (DEREALIZATION SECTION).

*67. When you experienced ______________________, (symptoms of depersonalization) were you having any other psychiatric problems, such as anxiety?

? (N) Y I

IF YES: What did your doctor say?

DESCRIBE:

*68. Do you have frequent episodes of anxiety or have you had panic attacks?

? N (Y) I

"The experience of depersonalization is often accompanied by considerable secondary anxiety, and frequently patients fear that their symptoms are a sign they are going 'insane'" (Nemiah 1989, p. 1042).

IF YES: What is your anxiety (or panic) like?

DESCRIBE: "Free-floating anxiety... sweating"

IF NO TO #68, GO TO #72 (PAGE 22).

IF SUBJECT HAS HAD SYMPTOMS OF ANXIETY DISORDER, RULE OUT ANXIETY SECONDARY TO DEPERSONALIZATION.

IF YES TO #68, ASK #69–#71:

*69. Are ______________________ (endorsed symptoms of anxiety disorder) related to your experiences of ______________________? (endorsed symptoms of depersonalization)

? N (Y) I

IF YES:

*70. In what way are they related? How often are they related?

- ☑ unclear
- ☐ not related
- ☐ sometimes related
- ☐ usually related

DESCRIBE:

*71. Do you usually feel

____
(endorsed symptoms of anxiety disorder)

first and then feel

______________________________,
(endorsed symptoms of depersonalization)

or is it the reverse?

Ratings

- ☐ unclear
- ☐ usually feels anxiety first
- ☐ sometimes feels anxiety first
- ☑ usually experiences depersonalization first

IF SUBJECT MEETS CRITERIA FOR DEPERSONALIZATION DISORDER, CONTINUE WITH #72.

IF SUBJECT DOES NOT MEET CRITERIA FOR DEPERSONALIZATION DISORDER, GO TO PAGE 25 (DEREALIZATION SECTION).

Rule Out Organic Etiology—Depersonalization

72. Just before you experienced

______________________________,
(endorsed symptoms of depersonalization)

were you using any drugs?

? (N) Y I

73. Were you drinking a lot?
(What did the doctor say?)

? (N) Y I

74. Did you have any trauma to your head that could have caused

______________________________?
(endorsed symptoms of depersonalization)

? (N) Y I

IF YES: Can you describe what occurred?

DESCRIBE:

? = inadequate information N = no Y = yes I = inconsistent information

75. Did you have any medical illness that could have caused

______________________________?
(endorsed symptoms of depersonalization)

? (N) Y I

IF YES: What medical illness did you have?

DESCRIBE:

IF YES TO #72, #73, #74, OR #75, ASK #76.
IF NO TO #72, #73, #74, AND #75, GO TO PAGE 25 (DEREALIZATION SECTION).

76. Have you ever experienced

____
(endorsed symptoms of depersonalization)

when you were not using

______________________________?
(substance or illness endorsed in #72–#75)

? N Y I

77. How often does that occur?
(Rate most frequent period.)

Frequency of Depersonalization

- ❐ unclear
- ❐ rarely (up to 4 isolated episodes)
- ❐ occasionally (up to 4 episodes per year)
- ❐ frequently (5 episodes or more per year)
- ❐ monthly episodes (up to 3 per month)
- ❐ daily or weekly episodes (4 or more per month)

*78.

Depersonalization Disorder Criterion D

? N Y I

D. The depersonalization experience does not occur exclusively during the course of another mental disorder, such as Schizophrenia, Panic Disorder, Acute Stress Disorder, or another Dissociative Disorder, and is not due to the direct physiological effects of a substance (e.g., a drug of abuse, a medication) or a general medical condition (e.g., temporal lobe epilepsy).

? = inadequate information N = no Y = yes I = inconsistent information

APPENDIX 4

Questions Often Asked About the SCID-D

The SCID-D appears to be an effective diagnostic instrument. Can I shorten the interview without affecting the integrity of the results?

The *Interviewer's Guide* specifies four permissible abbreviations of the interview, the last two of which are situational:

- Omission of questions marked with asterisks, which are intended to provide additional descriptive information but are not diagnostically discriminating for Dissociative Disorders
- Omission of questions in parentheses, if they are not relevant and/or the patient has already supplied sufficient information
- Omission of questions pertaining to substance abuse or the presence of medical illness, *if the subject has no history of either, as reported in the "Psychiatric History" section*
- Omission of the "Psychiatric History" section, *if that information has been previously obtained*

Refer to p. 40 of the *Interviewer's Guide* for a fuller explanation of these four items. However, further abbreviation of the SCID-D may affect the integrity of the results. If time constraints are at issue, it is advisable to administer the instrument over several sessions rather than to omit items or entire sections. Relevant considerations include the following:

- The distinctive symptom constellations that characterize the different Dissociative Disorders. Because each of the DSM-IV Dissociative Disorders has its own specific symptom profile, an interviewer who skips items or sections may miss the characteristic features of a given symptom as it manifests within the constellation of a specific Dissociative Disorder. Omissions may thus compromise the accuracy of the differential diagnosis.
- The nature of dissociative symptomatology and patient anxiety about symptom disclosure. Some manifestations of dissociation are difficult to describe; others may reflect the interconnection of the five core dissociative symptoms, such as when a person is amnestic for indications of identity alteration. SCID-D research indicates that it is not unusual for subjects to expand on their early endorsements of symptoms at later points in the interview. In addition, the pacing of the SCID-D is intended to allow the patient to answer questions in a relaxed and unhurried setting. Abbreviation of the instrument may hinder rapport and consequent full symptom disclosure.
- The consequences of misdiagnosis and inappropriate treatment. An interview requiring 2–3 hours is considerably more time efficient than years or decades of misdirected treatment.
- Forensic considerations. In the event of involvement with the legal system, it is a protection for the clinician if he or she has administered the SCID-D without unauthorized cuts or abbreviations.

I am interested in using the SCID-D in a clinical setting. How should I prepare myself to administer it appropriately?

- Familiarize yourself with the SCID-D and the *Interviewer's Guide.*

- Attend workshops for additional training. Further information about SCID-D workshops can be obtained by contacting the author.
- Begin by administering the SCID-D to patients who are cooperative and interested.
- If you are new to the field of dissociation or semistructured interviews, gain experience by administering the instrument one section at a time until you feel comfortable with all sections of it.
- Review *Handbook for the Assessment of Dissociation: A Clinical Guide* (Steinberg 1995).

To which of my patients should I administer the SCID-D?

Patients in any of the following categories are at higher risk for previously undetected Dissociative Disorders:

- Patients with a history of trauma and/or diagnosed with posttraumatic stress disorder
- Patients previously diagnosed as having "atypical" or "not otherwise specified" disorders
- Patients with a history of eating disorders or recurrent or atypical depression
- Patients who have been diagnosed with borderline personality disorder
- Patients who fall into one or more of the following categories: 1) patients whose symptoms meet criteria for more than two psychiatric diagnoses or who have a history of fluctuating symptoms leading to a variety of diagnoses; 2) patients who endorse hearing voices but are otherwise without symptoms of psychosis; 3) patients who have difficulty recalling symptom histories; or 4) patients who have a history of unsuccessful treatments with a series of therapists.

It is therefore advisable to consider administering the SCID-D to such patients.

I sometimes serve as an expert witness in the courtroom. What should I know about the SCID-D?

- The Summary Score Sheet of the SCID-D is designed to be filed with patient records and can be submitted in court as documentation. In addition, the interview booklet itself with the clinician's notes may be offered as evidence. This documentation may be particularly useful for expert witnesses testifying in regard to the use of hypnosis in a given case. For a fuller discussion of the applications of the SCID-D to hypnotherapy, please see the following question.
- SCID-D questions are phrased to avoid leading or intrusive wording. The open-ended format of the questions is intended to elicit free narrative recall of dissociative episodes, including spontaneous descriptions of past trauma.
- Certain categories of parties in civil or criminal cases should be routinely evaluated with the SCID-D for evidence of underlying Dissociative Disorders. These categories include 1) persons with a history of dissociative symptoms and/or posttraumatic stress disorder prior to arrest; 2) persons with a history of sexual addiction or sexual assault; 3) persons previously and/or currently diagnosed with schizophrenia or atypical psychosis (this population includes a statistical overrepresentation of violent offenders and persons found not guilty by reason of insanity; in addition, many persons with Dissociative Disorders are misdiagnosed as schizophrenic); 4) persons with a history of substance abuse; 5) persons with a history of recurrent suicidal or homicidal ideation or attempts; 6) persons with a history of self-mutilation or self-injury; and 7) persons who manifest dissociative symptoms following commission of a crime; depersonalization and other dissociated states commonly occur in persons who have committed particularly gruesome murders (Dietz 1992).
- The SCID-D can be repeatedly administered to a subject, by the same or by different interview-

ers, 1) to monitor changes in the severity of a suspect's symptomatology, 2) in cases involving a new consultant who wants to repeat the test, 3) in cases in which both prosecution and defense want to have the defendant evaluated by independent experts, 4) in controversial or contested cases in which either prosecution or defense wants to have the defendant evaluated by more than one expert to increase the reliability of the diagnosis, and 5) to assess the possibility of malingering. Although no diagnostic instrument is completely fool-proof against malingering, the SCID-D's semistructured format is designed to minimize the possibility of either "faking good" (defensiveness) or "faking bad" (malingering). In addition, it is difficult for malingerers to simulate Dissociative Identity Disorder for long periods (Kluft 1987b; Resnick 1984). According to Resnick (1984), "Extended interviews may be useful because unforced dissociation most often occurs between 2.5 and 4 hours after beginning an interview" (p. 43). The length of a full SCID-D interview may be helpful in discriminating between genuine and feigned dissociation.

I use hypnosis as an adjunct to psychotherapy. Should I administer the SCID-D to my patients?

It is recommended that therapists who use hypnosis as an adjunctive treatment modality administer the SCID-D before trance induction, for several reasons:

- The Summary Score Sheet allows for timely documentation of a patient's baseline symptomatology before hypnotic induction, thus allowing the clinician to distinguish between dissociative symptoms endorsed before hypnosis and those elicited as a result of hypnosis.
- The content or pattern of the patient's replies to SCID-D items may assist the practitioner in assessing the patient's hypnotizability and in selecting appropriate forms of trance induction.
- In some instances, the SCID-D may help to identify patients for whom hypnosis is contraindicated as a treatment modality.

Are there any contraindications to administration of the SCID-D?

The SCID-D can be administered over a series of shorter interview sessions if the patient has a short attention span, as may be the case with adolescents. Good results were obtained with adolescent patients when the instrument was administered in this way (Steinberg and Steinberg, in press [a]; Steinberg and Steinberg, in press [b]). However, other instances in which administration of the SCID-D is contraindicated include

- When the patient is agitated or uncooperative
- When the patient has not been stabilized (exhibits homicidal or suicidal ideation)
- When the patient is under the influence of drugs or alcohol
- When the patient requires immediate attention to medical conditions (e.g., patients with seizure disorder or anorexic patients requiring nutritional stabilization)
- When the patient is experiencing an acute reaction to recent trauma and cannot be attentive. If the clinician suspects that the patient has acute stress disorder, it is best to address the acute symptoms first and administer the SCID-D when the patient is able to be attentive.

In sum, interviewers should use good clinical judgment on a case-by-case basis and not administer the SCID-D in situations in which they would not administer other psychometric evaluations.

What should I tell the patient about the SCID-D prior to administration?

In cases in which the patient has been referred to you for a diagnostic evaluation, he or she will usually expect some type of formal assessment or interview. It will ordinarily be sufficient to explain the SCID-D as a specialized interview that will help to clarify the nature of his or her symptoms and may assist the referring therapist in treatment planning. You can also reassure the patient that he or she will have an opportunity to discuss the interview with you and that you will discuss the findings with the referring therapist.

When the SCID-D is administered during ongoing therapy with a patient you have identified as being at risk for a Dissociative Disorder, you can introduce the interview as a tool for helping your patient understand some of his or her symptoms better. If the patient seems apprehensive, you can add that the instrument does not have right or wrong answers but is open ended to allow for full description of his or her experiences. In addition, you can tell the patient that he or she will have an opportunity to discuss the results and that many people have found the feedback session to be an important step in their recovery process.

Most of my patients are members of minority groups and come from the inner city. Can I use the SCID-D with this patient population?

The SCID-D has been field-tested for cross-cultural validity in a wide variety of patient populations in the United States and Western Europe. Findings indicate that the five core dissociative symptoms as measured in the North American population are the same across racial and economic groups. The SCID-D's format is intended to allow the patient to describe his or her dissociative experiences in his or her own words and speech patterns. Items are worded at the sixth-grade level and can be understood by most adults—whatever their specific educational attainments or background. The SCID-D is being field-tested in a Spanish translation to meet the needs of clinicians serving Hispanic patients.

I don't belong to any particular "school" of psychotherapy. Does the SCID-D require knowledge of or commitment to any particular theoretical model?

The SCID-D is neutral with respect to the various models and traditions within psychotherapy. It can be used by psychoanalysts, family therapists, Jungians, cognitive therapists, or adherents of any other model of therapy, as well as by those who consider themselves eclectics.

I am a hospital administrator. What clinical settings should provide routine screening for Dissociative Disorders using the SCID-D?

Given the fact that certain patient subpopulations are at higher risk for undetected Dissociative Disorders, persons receiving treatment in the following settings should be evaluated with the SCID-D:

- Veterans Administration or military hospitals (patients who were in active combat or who have received the diagnosis of Posttraumatic Stress Disorder). SCID-D research indicates that a subset of patients with Posttraumatic Stress Disorder have undetected Dissociative Disorders.
- Rape crisis units.
- Trauma centers.
- Substance abuse treatment units.
- Eating disorder clinics.
- Sexual disorders (including sexual offenders).

I am a researcher. What areas of study can be investigated with the SCID-D?

- Prevalence studies of dissociative symptoms and disorders in certain populations: persons diagnosed with Posttraumatic Stress Disorder; prisoners, including juvenile offenders; the military; persons in high-stress occupations (police, paramedics, firefighters, etc.); survivors of family or community trauma; minority groups; women; adolescent, mid-life, geriatric groups; persons with physical disabilities; chronic psychiatric inpatients; socially stressed populations (homeless persons, persons with HIV, etc.)

- Studies of dissociative symptoms and disorders in patients with coexisting disorders: Affective Disorders; Anxiety Disorders and Obsessive-Compulsive Disorder; Attention-Deficit Disorders; Substance Use and Eating Disorders; Somatoform Disorders; Gender Identity Disorders; Sexual Disorders and Paraphilias; other addictions (sexual addictions, compulsive gambling, compulsive spending, compulsive religiosity, etc.); Factitious Disorders; Axis II Personality Disorders; seizure disorders, and/or pseudoseizures
- Epidemiological studies
- Longitudinal studies: families with intergenerational patterns of Dissociative Disorders; abusive families; studies of dissociative symptomatology across the life cycle
- Treatment and outcome studies: medication trials; comparisons of different forms of psychotherapy; comparisons of different treatment modalities
- Sociological and cross-cultural studies: comparisons of dissociative symptomatology in different cultures; comparisons of dissociative symptomatology in different socioeconomic groups

References

American Psychiatric Association: Diagnostic and Statistical Manual of Mental Disorders, 3rd Edition, Revised. Washington, DC, American Psychiatric Association, 1987

American Psychiatric Association: DSM-IV Options Book: Work in Progress 9/1/91. Washington, DC, American Psychiatric Association, 1991

American Psychiatric Association: Diagnostic and Statistical Manual of Mental Disorders, 4th Edition. Washington, DC, American Psychiatric Association, 1994

Bliss EL: Multiple personalities: a report of 14 cases with implications for schizophrenia and hysteria. Arch Gen Psychiatry 37:1388–1397, 1980

Bliss EL: Multiple personality, allied disorders and hypnosis. New York, Oxford University Press, 1986

Boon S, Draijer N: Diagnosing Dissociative Disorders in the Netherlands: a pilot study with the Structured Clinical Interview for DSM-III-R Dissociative Disorders. Am J Psychiatry 148:458–462, 1991

Brauer R, Harrow M, Tucker GJ: Depersonalization phenomena in psychiatric patients. Br J Psychiatry 117:509–515, 1970

Braun BG, Sachs RG: The development of Multiple Personality Disorder: predisposing, precipitating, and perpetuating factors, in Childhood Antecedents of Multiple Personality. Edited by Kluft RP. Washington, DC, American Psychiatric Press, 1985, pp 37–64

Bryer J, Nelson B, Miller J, et al: Childhood sexual and physical abuse as factors in adult psychiatric illness. Am J Psychiatry 144:1426–1430, 1987

Clary W, Burstin K, Carpenter J: Multiple Personality and Borderline Personality Disorder. Psychiatr Clin North Am 7:89–100, 1984

Coons P: The differential diagnosis of multiple personality: a comprehensive review. Psychiatr Clin North Am 7:51–67, 1984

Coons PM, Milstein V: Psychogenic amnesia: a clinical investigation of 25 cases. Dissociation 5(2):73–79, 1992

Coons P, Bowman E, Milstein V: Multiple Personality Disorder: a clinical investigation of 50 cases. J Nerv Ment Dis 176:519–527, 1988

Davison K: Episodic depersonalization: observations on 7 patients. Br J Psychiatry 110:505–513, 1964

Dietz PE: Mentally disordered offenders: patterns in the relationship between mental disorder and crime. Psychiatr Clin North Am 15:539–551, 1992

Dinges PR: Partial dissociation as encountered in the borderline patient. J Am Acad Psychoanal 5:327–334, 1977

Ellerstein N, Canavan J: Sexual abuse of boys. Am J Dis Child 134:250–257, 1980

Emslie G, Rosenfelt A: Incest reported by children and adolescents hospitalized for severe psychiatric problems. Am J Psychiatry 140:708–711, 1983

Endicott J, Spitzer RL: A diagnostic interview: the Schedule for Affective Disorders and Schizophrenia. Arch Gen Psychiatry 35:837–844, 1978

Endicott J, Spitzer RL, Fleiss JL, et al: The Global Assessment Scale: a procedure for measuring overall severity of psychiatric disturbance. Arch Gen Psychiatry 33:766–771, 1976

Fine CG: The cognitive sequelae of incest, in Incest-Related Syndromes of Adult Psychopathology. Edited by Kluft RP. Washington, DC, American Psychiatric Press, 1990, pp 161–182

Goff DC, Brotman AW, Kindlon D, et al: The delusion of possession in chronically psychotic patients. J Nerv Ment Dis 179:567–571, 1991

Goff DC, Olin JA, Jenike MA, et al: Dissociative symptoms in patients with Obsessive-Compulsive Disorder. J Nerv Ment Dis 180:332–337, 1992

Goodwin JM, Attias R: Eating disorders in survivors of multimodal childhood abuse, in Clinical Perspectives on Multiple Personality Disorder. Edited by Kluft RP, Fine CG. Washington, DC, American Psychiatric Press, 1993, pp 327–341

Greaves G: Multiple personality: 165 years after Mary Reynolds. J Nerv Ment Dis 168:577–596, 1980

Hall P, Steinberg M: Clinical applications of the SCID-D: first cases. (submitted for publication)

Hathaway SR, McKinley JC: Minnesota Multiphasic Personality Inventory, Revised. Minneapolis, University of Minnesota, 1970

Horevitz RP, Braun BG: Are multiple personalities borderline? Psychiatr Clin North Am 7:69–87, 1984

Husain A, Chapel J: History of incest in girls admitted to a psychiatric hospital. Am J Psychiatry 140:591–593, 1983

Kihlstrom JF: Dissociative and conversion disorders, in Cognitive Science and Clinical Disorders. Edited by Stein DJ, Young J. Orlando, FL, Academic Press, 1992

Kluft RP: An introduction to Multiple Personality Disorder. Psychiatric Annals 14:19–24, 1984

Kluft RP: The natural history of Multiple Personality Disorder, in Childhood Antecedents of Multiple Personality. Edited by Kluft RP. Washington, DC, American Psychiatric Press, 1985, pp 197–238

Kluft RP: An update on Multiple Personality Disorder. Hosp Community Psychiatry 38:363–372, 1987a

Kluft RP: The simulation and dissimulation of multiple personality disorder. Am J Clin Hypn 30:104–118, 1987b

Kluft RP: The Dissociative Disorders, in The American Psychiatric Press Textbook of Psychiatry. Edited by Talbott JA, Hales RE, Yudofsky SC. Washington, DC, American Psychiatric Press, 1988, pp 557–585

Kluft RP, Steinberg M, Spitzer R: DSM-III-R revisions in the Dissociative Disorders: an explanation of their observation and rationale. Dissociation 1(1):39–46, 1988

Lewis DO, Bard JS: Multiple personality and forensic issues. Psychiatr Clin North Am 14:750–756, 1991

Loewenstein MD, Hamilton J, Alagna S, et al: Experiential sampling in the study of Multiple Personality Disorder. Am J Psychiatry 144:19–24, 1987

Marcum JM, Wright K, Bissell WG: Chance discovery of Multiple Personality Disorder in a depressed patient by amobarbital interview. J Nerv Ment Dis 174:489–492, 1986

Myers M: Physical and sexual abuse histories of male psychiatric patients (letter). Am J Psychiatry 148:399, 1991

Nemiah JC: Dissociative Disorders (hysterical neurosis, dissociative type), in Comprehensive Textbook of Psychiatry/5, 5th Edition, Vol 1. Edited by Kaplan HI, Sadock BJ. Baltimore, MD, Williams & Wilkins, 1989, pp 1028–1044

Noyes J, Hoenk P, Kuperman S, et al: Depersonalization in accident victims and psychiatric patients. J Nerv Ment Dis 164:401–407, 1977

Putnam FW Jr: Dissociation as a response to extreme trauma, in Childhood Antecedents of Multiple Personality. Edited by Kluft RP. Washington, DC, American Psychiatric Press, 1985, pp 65–97

Putnam FW, Guroff JJ, Silberman EK, et al: The clinical phenomenology of Multiple Personality Disorder: review of 100 recent cases. J Clin Psychiatry 47:285–293, 1986

Raskin A, Schulterbrandt J, Reatig N, et al: Replication of factors of psychopathology in interview, ward behavior and self-report ratings of hospitalized depressives. J Nerv Ment Dis 148:87–98, 1969

Resnick P: The detection of malingered mental illness. Behavioral Sciences and the Law 2:21–37, 1984

Roberts WW: Normal and abnormal depersonalization. Journal of Mental Science 106:478–492, 1960

Rosenbaum M: The role of the term Schizophrenia in the decline of the diagnoses of multiple personality. Arch Gen Psychiatry 37:1383–1385, 1980

Rosenfeld A: Incidence of history of incest among 18 female psychiatric patients. Am J Psychiatry 136:791–795, 1979

Ross C, Norton G: Multiple Personality Disorder patients with a prior diagnosis of Schizophrenia. Dissociation 1:39–42, 1988

Sansonnet-Hayden H, Haley G, Marriage K, et al: Sexual abuse and psychopathology in hospitalized adolescents. J Am Acad Child Adolesc Psychiatry 26:753–757, 1987

Spiegel D: Dissociation and hypnosis in Posttraumatic Stress Disorders. Journal of Traumatic Stress 1:17–33, 1988

Spiegel D: Dissociation and trauma, in American Psychiatric Press Review of Psychiatry, Vol 10. Edited by Tasman A, Goldfinger SM. Washington, DC, American Psychiatric Press, 1991, pp 261–275

Spiegel D: The dissociative disorders, in The American Psychiatric Press Textbook of Psychiatry, 2nd Edition. Edited by Hales RE, Yudofsky SC, Talbott JA. Washington, DC, American Psychiatric Press, 1994, pp 633–652

Spiegel D, Cardeña E: Dissociative mechanisms in Posttraumatic Stress Disorder, in Posttraumatic Stress Disorder: Etiology, Phenomenology, and Treatment. Edited by Wolf ME, Mosnaim AD. Washington, DC, American Psychiatric Press, 1990, pp 22–34

Spiegel D, Rosenfeld A: Spontaneous hypnotic age regression: case report. J Clin Psychiatry 45:522–524, 1984

Spitzer RL, Williams JBW, Gibbon M, et al: Structured Clinical Interview for DSM-III-R (SCID). Washington, DC, American Psychiatric Press, 1990

Steinberg M: The Structured Clinical Interview for DSM-III-R Dissociative Disorders. New Haven, CT, Yale University School of Medicine, 1985

Steinberg M (principal investigator): Field trials of the Structured Clinical Interview for DSM-III-R Dissociative Disorders. New Haven, CT, Yale University School of Medicine, 1989–1992

Steinberg M: The spectrum of depersonalization: assessment and treatment, in American Psychiatric Press Review of Psychiatry, Vol 10. Edited by Tasman A, Goldfinger SM. Washington, DC, American Psychiatric Press, 1991, pp 223–247

Steinberg M: Interviewer's Guide to the Structured Clinical Interview for DSM-IV Dissociative Disorders (SCID-D), Revised Edition. Washington, DC, American Psychiatric Press, 1994a

Steinberg M: Structured Clinical Interview for DSM-IV Dissociative Disorders (SCID-D), Revised Edition. Washington, DC, American Psychiatric Press, 1994b

Steinberg M: Systematizing dissociation: symptomatology and diagnostic assessment, in Dissociation: Culture, Mind, and Body. Edited by Spiegel D. Washington, DC, American Psychiatric Press, 1994c, pp 59–88

Steinberg M: Handbook for the Assessment of Dissociation: A Clinical Guide. Washington, DC, American Psychiatric Press, 1995

Steinberg A, Steinberg M: Systematic assessment of multiple personality disorder in an adolescent who is blind. Dissociation (in press [a])

Steinberg M, Steinberg A: Systematic assessment of MPD in adolescents using the SCID-D: three case studies. Bull Menninger Clin (in press [b])

Steinberg M, Howland F, Cicchetti DV: The Structured Clinical Interview for DSM-III-R Dissociative Disorders: A Preliminary Report, in Proceedings of the International Conference on Multiple Personality and Dissociative States. Edited by Braun B. Chicago, IL, Rush Presbyterian Hospital, 1986

Steinberg M, Kluft RP, Coons PM, Bowman ES, Fine CG, Fink DL, Hall PE, Rounsaville BJ, Cicchetti DV: Multicenter field trials of the Structured Clinical Interview for DSM-IV Dissociative Disorders (SCID-D). New Haven, CT, Yale University School of Medicine, 1989–1993

Steinberg M, Rounsaville B, Cicchetti DV: The Structured Clinical Interview for DSM-III-R Dissociative Disorders: preliminary report on a new diagnostic instrument. Am J Psychiatry 147:76–82, 1990

Steinberg M, Rounsaville BJ, Cicchetti DV, et al: Distinguishing between schizophrenia and multiple personality disorder: a systematic evaluation of overlapping symptoms using a structured interview. J Nerv Ment Dis 182:495–500, 1994

Stern C: The etiology of multiple personalities. Psychiatr Clin North Am 7:149–160, 1984

Tasman A, Goldfinger SM (eds): American Psychiatric Press Review of Psychiatry, Volume 10. Washington, DC, American Psychiatric Press, 1991, 139–276

Terr L: Childhood traumas: an outline and overview. Am J Psychiatry 148:10–20, 1991

Torem M: Dissociative states presenting as eating disorders. Am J Clin Hypn 29:137–142, 1986

Trueman D: Depersonalization in a nonclinical population. J Psychol 116:107–112, 1984

Wilbur C: Multiple personality and child abuse. Psychiatr Clin North Am 7:3–8, 1984